The Practitioner as Assessor

Education Centre Library
Southend Hospital, Prittlewell Chase,
Westcliff-on-Sea, Essex SS0 0RY
Tel: (Tel: 01702 385090
or ext 5090

KT-406-338

WITHDRAWN
FROM STOCK

2

1 4 JLF 2012

209560

For Baillière Tindall:

Commissioning Editor: Susan Young
Project Development Manager: Dinah Thom
Project Manager: Ailsa Laing
Designer: Judith Wright
Illustrator: Daniel Grice

The Practitioner as Assessor

Sue Howard MA RGN RHV DNCert CertEd DNT

Acting Assistant Director (Education), Royal College of Nursing, London, UK

Anne Eaton BSc RCNT CertEd RNT RM RGN, D32,33,34,35, and 36

Education/VQ Adviser, Royal College of Nursing, London, UK

Foreword by

Roswyn Hakesley-Brown

Former President of the Royal College of Nursing, London, UK

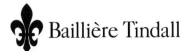 Baillière Tindall

EDINBURGH LONDON NEW YORK PHILADELPHIA ST LOUIS SYDNEY TORONTO 2003

BAILLIÈRE TINDALL
An imprint of Elsevier Science Limited

© 2003, Elsevier Science Limited. All rights reserved.

The right of Sue Howard and Anne Eaton to be identified as authors of this work has been asserted by them in accordance with the Copyright, Designs and Patents Act 1988

No part of this publication may be reproduced, stored in a retrieval system, or transmitted in any form or by any means, electronic, mechanical, photocopying, recording or otherwise, without either the prior permission of the publishers or a licence permitting restricted copying in the United Kingdom issued by the Copyright Licensing Agency, 90 Tottenham Court Road, London W1T 4LP. Permissions may be sought directly from Elsevier's Health Sciences Rights Department in Philadelphia, USA. Phone: (+1) 215 238 7869, fax: (+1) 215 238 2239, e-mail: healthpermissions@elsevier.com. You may also complete your request on-line via the Elsevier Science homepage (http://www.elsevier.com), by selecting 'Customer Support' and then 'Obtaining Permissions'.

First published 2003

ISBN 0 7020 2660 3

British Library Cataloguing in Publication Data
A catalogue record for this book is available from the British Library

Library of Congress Cataloging in Publication Data
A catalog record for this book is available from the Library of Congress

Notice
Medical knowledge is constantly changing. Standard safety precautions must be followed, but as new research and clinical experience broaden our knowledge, changes in treatment and drug therapy may become necessary or appropriate. Readers are advised to check the most current product information provided by the manufacturer of each drug to be administered to verify the recommended dose, the method and duration of administration, and contraindications. It is the responsibility of the practitioner, relying on experience and knowledge of the patient, to determine dosages and the best treatment for each individual patient. Neither the Publisher nor the authors assume any liability for any injury and/or damage to persons or property arising from this publication.

The Publisher

your source for books, journals and multimedia in the health sciences
www.elsevierhealth.com

The publisher's policy is to use **paper manufactured from sustainable forests**

Printed in China

Contents

To my Mum and Dad, Stephen, Caroline and Daniel for their everlasting belief in me.

SH

To Roger, Katie and Gemma for supporting me. Thank you.

AE

Foreword

Education is essential for the development of expert nurses and other health care practitioners, in order for them to be able to deliver the high quality care that patients need, expect and deserve. The role of the assessor is fundamental to this crucial process. Who better to carry out this important function than the expert practitioners themselves? This text offers a valuable resource not only for aspiring assessors, but also for anyone else who finds themselves in the privileged position of developing and supporting new generations of health care providers; be they nurses, health care assistants or members of other health care disciplines. Additionally, the people who are being assessed will benefit from the wise insights that can be gained from this book.

Making judgements about fitness for practice and purpose is not a responsibility to be taken lightly. However, these judgements have to be made with integrity and rigour, given that the need for health care professionals who are not only highly competent, but also caring and compassionate, has never been so great.

This serious assessment responsibility also has to be viewed against a complex backdrop of increasing public expectations, competing policy imperatives, the shifting paradigms from case management to public health agendas and radically changing relationships such as from passive patients to patient partnerships. Alongside this challenging health care landscape is the need to be able to assess the integration of theoretical excellence with clinical competence. This sensitive combining of the 'how?' and the 'why?' is the essence of modern health care. The days when I, as a student nurse, was told that I was not paid to think when asking challenging questions, are thankfully long since past!

Just as I believe passionately in the rights of patients in accessing high quality care delivered by expertly prepared practitioners, I also believe in the rights of health care professionals to fair and constructive assessment. This book should facilitate exactly that. It should also promote the dissemination of good practice, as well as affording the expert practitioner the opportunity to reflect on their own practice. Continuing professional development, encapsulated within an ethos of lifelong learning, should not preclude the utilisation of feedback in both directions in the assessor–assessee relationship. This book should enable us to have that and to put our reflective practice commitment into our quality care repertoire.

Demonstrating effective leadership through good assessment practices also makes a major contribution to the development of leaders of the future as they move incrementally up the skills escalator. The power of positive role models should never be underestimated in the patient care scheme of things. The 'do as you would be done by' philosophy is a key element in caring for the carers. Cascading confidence, where appropriate, produces unanticipated dividends for both patients and the health care team. It is important to nurture the feel-good factor in the interests of all stakeholders in the health care endeavour. Identifying and tackling weaknesses, as well as celebrating achievements, is a high-level skill which this book will help to cultivate.

Implicit in the assessment process is the requirement that practice be evidenced-based. The demands that this can place on the assessment relationship are enormous and need to be handled with dexterity and knowledge, in order to promote the development of autonomous clinical decision-making. Using critically evaluated evidence to underpin decisions surrounding such issues as risk management, planning/coordinating care and evaluating outcomes is a sophisticated process requiring similarly sophisticated assessment procedures in order to ascertain competence. Expert practitioners are the individuals who have reached this level of sophistication and should be acknowledged and rewarded for the valuable resource that they undoubtedly provide. But they, in their turn, need the support that this book can provide.

Work-based learning is in the ascendancy. Those who are responsible for assessment are gatekeepers, in every sense of the word, to the world of fully-fledged, high quality professional practice. Using the right tools to carry out this important task not only emancipates the assessor, it ensures the integrity of the legitimisation of knowledge-based competence that tells the patient that this particular health care professional really knows his or her stuff. Confident staff means confident patients and that can only be good news for health care delivery in the UK and we need good assessor leaders to achieve this.

An old Chinese proverb notes that we need to:

> Go to the people
> Live among them
> Start with what they have
> Build with them
> And when the deed is done
> The mission accomplished
> Of the best leadership
> The people will say
> We have done it ourselves

This book will help all assessors to do this with some authenticity and authority. Enjoy the journey... Bon Voyage!

University of Glamorgan 2003   **Roswyn Hakesley-Brown**

Preface

The writing of this book has stemmed from two key events: the refocusing of nursing as a practice-based profession and the need for nurses at all levels to understand the principles underpinning – and the factors involved in – the assessment of nurses and nursing in the practice setting.

The interrelationship between the assessment of theory and of practice is clearly understood and it is our conscious intention to focus on practice assessment. This is because, firstly, the theoretical aspects of teaching and assessing in nursing practice have been very ably written about elsewhere (*see* Nicklin & Kenworthy 2000). Secondly, we wished to write a book that would act as a resource guide for any practitioner who, at whatever stage in their career, is involved in the assessment of students in practice, whether they be pre- or postregistration or health care assistants. The book's purpose is to reflect the new focus on outcomes and competencies as a method of ensuring fitness for practice.

Although practice assessment is only one part of the wider picture of assessment, it is sometimes helpful to break it down into its component parts. This enables the issues surrounding practice assessment to be more readily understood, and applied to the situations we as nurses often find ourselves in when faced with supporting students in practice.

This book is for all mentors, assessors, nurses, students or health care assistants working in various situations – whether it be in hospitals, patients' homes, clinics, health centres, nursing homes, prisons or voluntary organisations – who want to know more about assessing nurses and nursing in practice.

Because the book looks at the elements of and the principles underpinning the assessment of practice, it may also be useful to other allied health professionals who have student assessment as a part of their role.

In recent years, nurses involved in the assessment of practice have held titles of mentor, assessor or both, while in terms of VQ assessment the term assessor has been used. The term mentor is used to denote the role of the nurse, midwife or health visitor who facilitates learning and supervises and assesses students in the practice setting (ENB & DoH 2001, p. 9). For the purpose of this book the terms mentor/assessor will therefore be used interchangeably.

The first chapter of the book contextualises assessment in relation to the nursing and health care strategies of England, Northern Ireland, Scotland and Wales. Chapter 2 illustrates the work of the UKCC (now Nursing and Midwifery Council) enquiry into nursing education. Chapters 3–6 provide the 'how to' of the assessment process. While these chapters fit together under the umbrella of assessment in practice, they could equally be explored in isolation. Chapters 3–6 also contain exercises, which allow for reflection and the opportunity to assess your personal understanding of the content.

We hope you find the book useful.

REFERENCES

English National Board for Nursing, Midwifery and Health Visiting & Department of Health (ENB & DoH) 2001 Preparation of Mentors and Teachers: A new framework for guidance. English National Board, London

Nicklin PJ, Kenworthy N (eds) 2000 Teaching and Assessing in Nursing Practice: An Experiential Approach, 3rd Edn. Baillière Tindall, London

London 2003   Anne Eaton
                                                                   Sue Howard

1 National nursing strategies and their impact on practice

INTRODUCTION

Assessment of clinical skills, and the competence to perform safely in practice lies at the heart of nursing, regardless of who delivers nursing care, and where that care is delivered. Assessment is an integral part of professional nursing programmes, whether they are at preregistration level or part of continuing professional development. It also forms a significant aspect of nurses' responsibilities not only within nursing itself but also with other providers of care. This is demonstrated in the development of non-professional carers supporting registered nurses in patient/client care, through National Vocational Qualifications (NVQs) and Scottish Vocational Qualifications (SVQs).

A number of major developments have been paramount in changing the focus and direction of nursing, both from a strategic and an operational level all of which ultimately impact on the process of assessment.

The aim of this chapter is to highlight the governmental strategies responsible for this, and identify the impact these documents have had, and will have, on all individuals delivering nursing care, however far removed they may at first appear.

LEARNING OBJECTIVES

After reading this chapter, you should be able to:

◆ outline the four nursing strategy documents

◆ identify key issues respective to your own country of employment

◆ compare the similarities and differences between the strategies of the four countries.

AN OVERVIEW OF NURSING STRATEGIES

It is becoming increasingly commonplace for the four countries of the UK to devise and develop their own processes and strategies in relation to how health care is organised and delivered. This ultimately will have an impact on nursing.

Northern Ireland was the first of the four countries to produce a nursing strategy: *Valuing diversity – a way forward, a strategy for nursing, midwifery and health visiting* (DHSS 1998). The Welsh strategy, *Realising the potential, a strategic framework for nursing, midwifery and health visiting in Wales into the 21st century* (NAW 1999) was published in July 1999, closely followed by the English strategy *Making a difference: strengthening the nursing, midwifery and health visiting contribution to health and health care* (DoH 1999a) in August of that year. This was published immediately prior to the United Kingdom Central Council for Nursing, Midwifery and Health Visiting (UKCC) Education Commission document *Fitness for practice* released in September 1999. The UKCC publication is a UK-wide document, covering all four countries. It is an important document that is closely related to the strategies outlined here and will be discussed in Chapter 2. Scotland was the last of the UK countries to produce a strategy: *Caring for Scotland: the strategy for Nursing and Midwifery in Scotland* (SEHD 2001) was published in March 2001.

It is important to note that the UKCC was replaced by the Nursing and Midwifery Council (NMC) on 1 April 2002. As a result, the book refers to work undertaken by the UKCC before this date and the NMC after it.

KEY POINTS FROM THE NORTHERN IRELAND STRATEGY

This section is based on *Valuing Diversity* (DHSS 1998). The outcomes of the strategy include:

- reshaping the profession to prepare for the future
- the need for strong leadership, both clinical and managerial
- the need to respond to increasing public expectations and demands for health and social care within limited resources
- greater emphasis on public health and community development
- working in partnership as part of multiprofessional teams.

It is worth remembering that this document was developed prior to the United Kingdom Central Council Education Commission document *Fitness for practice* (UKCC 1999) discussed in Chapter 2 and as a result does not provide in-depth information regarding specific developments in nursing education.

Clinical workforce issues

This part of the document identifies the need for a balance of skills in the nursing workforce, and states that 'vocational trained support workers are crucial to the provision of care to patients and clients.' Further, it states that 'nurses, midwives and health visitors must ensure that they are involved with the recruitment and assessment of vocationally trained support workers ... supervising their practice, assessing their competence' (DHSS 1998, p. 17).

Part 4 of the document refers to the issue of education. It recognises the need for nursing education to meet the changing needs of patients, clients and carers, and to be set within the strategic context of health care delivery, assessment, therefore, being seen as crucial to the development of the future workforce.

The need for lifelong learning is identified within the document, and it is argued that education will empower practitioners. The document notes that 'pre- and postregistration curricula must include objectives related to themes such as: clinical effectiveness; the promotion of health and wellbeing in communities, groups and individuals; commissioning at all levels and the development of specialist practitioner roles' (DHSS 1998, p. 23).

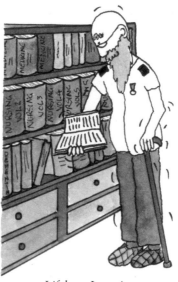

Lifelong Learning

You may be able to assess whether these themes have been incorporated into the preregistration curriculum in Northern Ireland after reviewing the UKCC's work on preregistration programmes outlined in Chapter 2.

KEY POINTS FROM THE WELSH STRATEGY

The Welsh strategy, *Realising the potential – a strategic framework for nursing, midwifery and health visiting in Wales into the 21st century* (NAW 1999), identifies in common with the strategies of the other three countries that the patient rather than the professions must be at the heart of developments in health care. The strategic goal of the document, and therefore the National Assembly for Wales and the whole profession, is 'to realise the full potential of nursing, midwifery and health visiting in order to meet, in collaboration with others, the future health needs of people in Wales' (NAW 1999, p. 16).

This strategy highlights the fact that nurses, midwives and health visitors are the largest single profession working in the NHS in Wales, and quantifies the number as more than 30,000. This indicates not only the size of the nursing, midwifery and health visiting workforce within the UK (the Nursing and Midwifery Council (NMC) has upwards of 650,000 registrants) but also the levels of support required to accommodate learning in practice.

Unlike the other strategies, the Welsh strategy makes a firm statement about the level of education required by nurses, midwives and health visitors, suggesting that because these groups work alongside medical colleagues they should receive the same level of education as these other health related professions. It reinforces the notion of graduate status, suggesting this is the level needed to underpin the cognitive skills required for critical analysis, problem solving, decision making and clinical judgement. It also identifies, however, the need to ensure that this exit level must not inhibit broad recruitment. The document introduces the idea of the inclusion of core skills in communication, the use of information technology, numeracy and so on (known as key skills from the NVQ perspective).

The document highlights the future development of the professions within Wales, suggesting the development of a 'distinctive identity' whilst 'remaining firmly within the family of nursing, midwifery and health visiting throughout the UK and the rest of the world.' (NAW 1999, p. 7)

The document states that 'the education of nurses, midwives and health visitors at all levels must take account of the changing environment of care. Education must continue to prepare practitioners who are fit for purpose, fit for practice and fit for award.' (NAW 1999, p. 11)

Implicit in this is the notion of professional accountability and the document cited the notion of professional competence in relation to new roles, as well as the need for delegation to 'properly trained' personnel, again emphasising the importance of assessment.

As with the strategy for Northern Ireland, when this strategy was written, the UKCC had yet to publish *Fitness for practice* (UKCC 1999) or develop the outcomes and competencies for preregistration programmes.

The Welsh strategy initiated a debate in relation to the potential benefits of generalist preregistration preparation, as opposed to the specific branch programmes of adult, child, learning disability and mental health at preregistration level currently in place. This issue is under review by the Nursing and Midwifery Council (NMC).

As identified in the English strategy, the Welsh strategy confirms the need to retain a competent workforce by 'the maintenance of close liaisons between education and service.' (NAW 1999, p. 12)

Since the publication of the Welsh nursing strategy, further work has continued and has led to the publication of a briefing paper *Creating the potential* (NAW 2000). Its purpose is to build on the strategy and provide a clear direction for the development and provision of professional education in Wales.

The briefing paper is intended to be a working document, which will assist both education and service providers in developing initiatives. The document sets out four principles which highlight and define the way forward.

ACHIEVING FITNESS FOR PRACTICE, PURPOSE AND AWARD

Principle 1 notes that fitness for practice is the responsibility of the appropriate regulatory body. In nursing this is the role of the NMC. The principle goes on to state that 'Preregistration education must produce a safe and competent practitioner who can demonstrate the competencies specified by statute and can be held accountable for his or her decisions and actions.' (NAW 2000, p. 15).

The principle identifies nursing as a practice-based profession, and 'clinical competence is as important as, and should be valued as highly as, theoretical excellence.' (NAW 2000, p. 15) Building on some of the issues around the definition of competence (see Chapter 3), Principle 1 also states that 'existing and future practitioners need to be able to make the best use of the range of skills and knowledge which they have developed as new roles and organisational structures emerge.' (NAW 2000, p. 15).

DEVELOPMENT AND LEADERSHIP OF PRACTICE AND EDUCATION

Principle 2 identifies that the professions of nursing, midwifery and health visiting need strong leaders, and defines lifelong learning as a professional responsibility. However, it also suggests that in order to facilitate such initiatives resources need to be made available. The principle is further strengthened by stating that 'nurses, midwives and health visitors should have the same opportunities and entitlements to protected time for continuing professional development as other professionals.' (NAW 2000, p. 17).

EXPANDING THE RESEARCH AND EDUCATION ENVIRONMENT

Principle 3 re-states the issue of the academic level of preregistration programmes and the need for them to be at the same level for all members of the multiprofessional health care team, i.e. graduate entry into practice. The principle recommends the expansion of multidisciplinary learning, and that the skills and knowledge that all staff can bring to patient/client care should be recognised. The principle identifies that research as a means of testing knowledge, and teaching as a means of transmitting knowledge, are paramount in the development of nursing skills and knowledge.

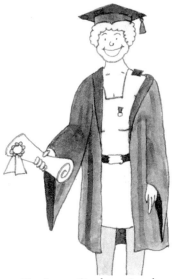

Moving to Graduate Level

MEETING FUTURE HUMAN RESOURCE REQUIREMENTS

Principle 4 reinforces the necessity for education to meet the needs of health services, reflecting the multiple places where care is delivered, and the needs of society for qualified nurses, midwives and health visitors. It argues the need for workforce development and planning, and data collection, stating that these are areas for current attention. Implicit in this is the need for robust systems that will identify the numbers of students who leave preregistration programmes before they have completed the course and their reasons for doing so.

Present and future needs

It is acknowledged within the document that current preparatory programmes for nurses, midwives and health visitors will take practice well into the new millennium. The World Health Organization Strategy for Nurse Education (WHO 2000) proposes that nurses, midwives and health visitors must be educated and trained to meet the challenges posed by:

- a new emphasis on health promotion and disease prevention
- community development
- multidisciplinary team working
- the provision of health services closer to where people work
- equality of access.

It could be argued that the UK is one of the leaders in this area, for example in the development of NHS Direct, Health Action Zones, and Walk-in Centres, which are often managed by nurses.

Fitness for practice

Creating the potential supports the notion of fitness for practice. This involves:

- autonomous clinical decision making

- personal accountability for decisions and actions.

Fitness for practice is not limited to the care of the physically sick in hospital or to the performance of tasks, but also includes:

- working with individuals

- working with families and communities

- assessment

- risk management

- planning care

- co-ordinating care

- evaluating outcomes

- delegation to, and supervision of, the work of assistants.

For the purpose of this book, the final bullet point on delegation must also incorporate the assessment of the competence of this workforce, especially in line with the *Code of professional conduct* (NMC 2002). This states in Section 4.2 'you are expected to work co-operatively within teams and to respect the skills, expertise and contributions of others', and in Section 6.4, 'you have a duty to facilitate students of nursing and midwifery and others to develop their competence'.

Fitness for purpose

The phrase 'fitness for purpose' represents the particular requirements of the employers, and their needs for specific roles and functions within health care delivery in all its forms. The strategy therefore suggests fitness for purpose must make sure that nurses, midwives and health visitors have the necessary *skills, knowledge and attitudes* to deliver the services that patients, clients and their families expect. Implicit in this is the notion of competence (discussed in Chapter 3).

This is supported by the *Code of professional conduct* (NMC 2002) which states that 'as a registered nurse or midwife, you must:

- protect and support the health of individual patients and clients
- protect and support the health of the wider community
- act in such a way that justifies the trust and confidence the public has in you
- uphold and enhance the good reputation of the professions.'

Fitness for award

Fitness for award is identified as the requirement of the higher education institutions that students achieve the level of attainment specified for a particular award to be given. This definition shows that the requirement extends beyond the professional sphere, and encompasses all who are undertaking an award, whether it be a nursing student within a university, or a health care assistant undertaking an S/NVQ through one of the awarding bodies – City and Guilds, Edexcel /Institute of Health Care Development (IHCD) and Scottish Qualifications Agency (SQA).

This quality assurance mechanism is further extended to such organisations as the Quality Assurance Agency (QAA) in respect of higher education institutions, and the Qualifications and Curriculum Authority (QCA) and Scottish Qualifications Authority (SQA) in respect of S/NVQs.

The document notes that preregistration education will in the future be based on defined competencies. This work has already been implemented throughout the UK following the development of the UKCC outcomes and competencies for preregistration nursing education. 'It is important to recognise that for professional practice … the definition of competency is broader than that specified for vocational training, and must include the intellectual competencies required for clinical decision making' (NAW 2000, p. 10).

KEY POINTS FROM THE ENGLISH STRATEGY

Making a difference (DoH 1999a) was distributed immediately before the dissemination of the UKCC's *Fitness for practice* (UKCC 1999). The strategy refers to the sharing of plans by the Government and the UKCC Commission to improve nursing education and training, thus emphasising the need for partnership between the two.

The remit of the document is vast as it incorporates the whole Government agenda for modernising the National Health Service, and covers many areas that are distinct from, but linked to, nursing education. For the purpose of this discussion, we will concentrate on Chapter 4, *Strengthening education and training*, which has an immediate impact upon nursing education in England.

Within this chapter, the Prime Minister, Tony Blair, identifies the need for 'a modern flexible system that enables and encourages people with different backgrounds and qualifications to acquire nursing skills and competencies in a flexible fashion.' This illustrates the partnership approach needed between higher education institutions and the NHS, which both have a commitment to prepare the professions and the need for 'practitioners who are fit for purpose, with excellent skills, and the knowledge and ability to provide the best care possible in the modern NHS.' (DoH 1999a, p. 23).

An issue not addressed within this national strategy, nor in the others, is the fact that up to 25% of qualified nurses work outside of the NHS. For example, they may work in the private and independent sectors, in a variety of settings, ranging from nursing homes, private hospitals, and industry. Wherever professional nurses and indeed non-professional carers are employed, they need the support of a rigorous assessment process and experienced and committed assessors.

Within the nursing strategy for England, the Government identifies one of the priorities as being the need to increase the level of practical skills within the training programmes and to provide more flexible career pathways into and within nursing and midwifery education.

The document suggests that individuals will benefit from more flexible approaches to education and training. One aim is to strengthen the links between vocational training and preregistration education, and subsequently to enable people working as health care assistants who wish to move into nursing or midwifery if they have the ability to do so.

'Fast tracking' as a process of crediting prior learning is introduced in the document (DoH 1999a, page 25), implying that a shortened route to registered nurse status be developed for people with the appropriate vocational qualifications.

The vital nature of practice placements in relation to the education process and the assessment of skills and competence taking place in these areas are also highlighted. Early exposure of nursing students to practical placements is seen as key to this: 'we want higher quality and longer placements in a genuinely supportive learning environment' (DoH 1999a, p. 27).

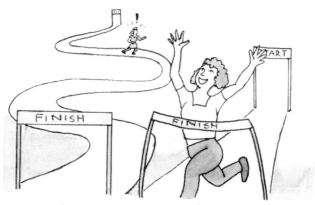

Shorter Routes to Registered Nurse Status

The document recognises and acknowledges the input and expertise needed to support students in practice, and suggests the importance of nurses being taught by those with recent practical experience of nursing. Since this proposal was made, many universities, often in partnership with their local NHS Trust, have developed new roles of 'practice facilitators' or 'practice educators'. These evolving roles, however, appear to be disparate and may not directly relate to students, but to the mentors and assessors who support students. There is a proposal that the Government wishes to enhance the status of those who provide practice-based learning. How this will happen is as yet undecided, but it is closely linked to clinical governance and the implementation of the recommendations within the English nursing strategy.

Targets set by the document state that from 1999 the Government expects to recruit 19,000 students onto nursing and midwifery programmes. This number will undoubtedly lead to an added burden on the practice-based staff who support and assess the clinical competence of this large group of learners.

Within the area of continuing professional development (CPD) the strategy identifies a need to expand and focus upon multidisciplinary learning, and cites reflection and experience as a means to achieving this. Again, the need for supervision and assessment becomes evident within this proposal. Ways of adequately meeting the need for assessment will be reviewed later.

'Developing a modern career framework' within the document introduces the potential for a new career structure, replacing clinical grades. The framework identifies a career trajectory, from health care assistant to consultant practitioner. The pathway suggests that movement within careers can happen as a lateral move as well as an upward progression. The peak of this trajectory will encompass the nurse consultant posts. The aim of this is to keep nurses at the forefront of care delivery.

This development in England has clear links to the Government's work on redefining pay structures and work roles, known as *Agenda for change*

(DoH 1999b). This is currently being debated throughout the UK and will potentially affect all health care professions, not just nurses. The process will include a process of job evaluation. The document states that 'we will work with professional organisations and trades unions and then UK Health Departments to develop clear statements of competence identifying the thresholds for each range.' (DoH 1999b, p. 34). The suggestion is that NHS employers will need to develop more detailed competency frameworks. This is mentioned here as it highlights another way in which competence and competencies can impact upon the health care workforce.

KEY POINTS FROM THE SCOTTISH STRATEGY

This section discusses *Caring for Scotland: the strategy for nursing and midwifery in Scotland* (SEHD 2001). This publication was the last of the four nursing strategies to be launched. The opening sentence by Susan Deacon, MSP, then Minister for Health and Community Care, states that 'Scotland is justifiably proud of its nurses and midwives.' The strategy outlines plans to build on this pride and 'points to the immense academic and personal challenges that becoming a nurse or midwife bring.' Furthermore, Anne Jarvie, Chief Nursing Officer in the Scottish Executive Health Department, suggests in her introduction that 'there has never been a better time to be a nurse or midwife in Scotland.'

The initiatives contained within the strategy bring together a number of previous publications and policies, such as *Towards a healthier Scotland* (SODoH 1999), and the new health plan for Scotland, *Our national health: a plan for action, a plan for change* (SEHD 2000).

Caring for Scotland centres on a number of themes, namely:

- the context in which policy is developed

- nursing and midwifery in Scotland: identifying and expanding on issues around meeting challenges of the key policy initiatives

- the vision – a window on the future: demonstrating and illustrating how nurses and midwives can build upon initiatives and involve the development of new and expanded roles

- rhetoric into reality: expanding upon issues related to accountability, leadership, professional development, career development, research and evidence based practice, and education

- delivering the vision: noting that the Scottish Executive has embarked upon a major programme to modernise NHS Scotland, and outlining the way in which nurses and midwives will enable this aim to become reality.

For the purpose of this chapter, the issues discussed are in relation to education. However, it is necessary to highlight that all areas relate to the vision for health care in Scotland which identifies the need for new skills and competence to enable the development of new and expanded roles. Clearly these competencies first need to be developed and then assessed.

Caring for Scotland reminds its readers that nurses are accountable to the NMC and that ultimately the NMC is accountable to the public, through the State; in this context the State being the Westminster Parliament.

The document makes a clear link between the issue of accountability and the development of clinical governance, which was introduced into Scotland in 1997, following the publication of *Designed to Care* (SODoH 1997). It identifies that a number of key requirements are needed in order to meet the clinical governance agenda, namely:

- staff must exercise accountability within frameworks laid down by professional regulatory bodies
- continuous quality improvement is the goal of the service
- continuing professional development is a key feature of the service
- clinical risk is identified and managed
- problems and complaints are used to promote learning and improve practice
- poor performance is recognised and actions taken to improve it.

In relation to the points above, the Scottish Executive reminds all nurses that it is their individual responsibility to ensure that they understand issues of accountability in relation to their clinical function, and in line with the UKCC documents *The code of professional conduct* (UKCC 1992a), and *The scope of professional practice* (UKCC 1992b). These two documents were replaced by the *Code of professional conduct* in June 2002 (NMC 2002). The Executive along with the NHS boards and professional organisations and unions will in turn ensure that the guidelines and arrangements for clinical governance reflect issues of individual accountability.

Clinical supervision is seen as the process by which the effective support of individuals can be achieved, and therefore the document calls upon all individual nurses and their employers to meet the requirements of clinical supervision. It reminds all concerned that, in order to do this, sufficient time and resources must be in place.

In line with the recommendations in *Fitness for practice* (UKCC 1999), *Caring for Scotland* sees support and clinical supervision of newly qualified staff as imperative if they are to develop in their chosen roles, and indeed, stay in the profession. The Scottish Executive sees the UKCC's recommendations regarding Post Registration Education and Practice (PREP) as integral to the notion of support in the immediate postregistration period. An aim, therefore, of the Executive in 2001 was to establish a Working Group who would consider the best way to support newly qualified nurses during their initial period of employment in the NHS within Scotland.

An additional purpose of the Working Group was to establish common standards based on good practice in order to support newly qualified nurses. In addition to this the NHS boards and Local Health Care Cooperatives (LHCCs) will provide a system of structured support for newly qualified nurses at a local level, in accordance with the common standards.

The document highlights that support workers are valued members of the multidisciplinary team in both hospital and community settings, especially in their support of nurses in caring for patients. The Scottish Executive therefore recognises the need for the accreditation of programmes of training and assessment to ensure that support workers are able to deliver care to a comparable high standard both safely and effectively.

The implication of this is that nurses are appropriately placed to lead this training and to supervise these workers in practice settings. The use of Scottish Vocational Qualifications (SVQs) is recognised in this context, as is the role of registered nurses in the delivery and assessment of these awards. However, the Scottish Executive expands on this concept by recommending that organisations need to recognise the resource implications of enabling nurses to train, assess, delegate and supervise the increasing numbers of support workers. The action the Executive expects is the development of a framework for the training, support and supervision of support workers and for Directors of Nursing to agree occupational standards for support workers.

The document reviews and reinforces the need for the development of leaders in the profession and acknowledges that ward sisters and charge nurses are already leaders who make vital inputs to the development of junior staff. The document also recognises further developments in this area, especially in line with the new posts of consultant nurses. However, the assertion that leadership does not have to equate with seniority in a clinical or management role will reassure some readers.

The recommendations include a review of current positions in respect of the accessibility and uptake of leadership programmes, and for a variety of bodies to ensure that leadership skills training programmes address identified unmet needs.

The Scottish Executive states that ward sisters and charge nurses must be empowered by their employers to deliver patient care and demonstrate clinical leadership. They must also have access to education and training, and managerial support to enable them to do their jobs, as well as to develop their roles in all aspects. Subsequently, the strategy recommends that all ward sisters and charge nurses have access to leadership development opportunities within their organisations.

The Scottish Executive views Continuing Professional Development (CPD) as paramount not only in ensuring quality patient care and developing staff but also in playing a major role in the recruitment and retention of staff. CPD is therefore seen as encompassing career development and advice, and the recognition that this can be sideways as well as upwards. Importance is placed on the need for career development options to utilise the talents of all nurses, freeing up their potential to reshape patient services.

The notion of career development applies to all staff, and the document includes support workers in this, recommending that clear career opportunities within nursing should also be available to support workers.

The document recognises that some NHS boards have used Scottish Vocational Qualifications (SVQs) at levels 2 and 3 to develop support workers, and this may enable them to enter preregistration nursing education programmes. The Scottish Qualifications Authority (SQA) and the National Board for Nursing, Midwifery and Health Visiting for Scotland (NBS), in conjunction with colleges of further education, have all worked together to develop a Higher National Certificate in Care that may be used to seek academic credit for the first year of preregistration nurse education.

A related recommendation is that support workers must be enabled to acquire a named award to at least SVQ level 2.

As with the English nursing strategy, *Making a difference* (DoH 1999a), and *Fitness for practice* (UKCC 1999), the Scottish Executive recognises the need to award academic and practice credit to nursing students who have to leave their preregistration programmes before the end. To this end, a further recommendation is that consideration be given to employment opportunities within NHS Scotland for students who do not complete the full 3-year programme.

These and other similar recommendations demand thorough assessment processes that are well documented, transparent and transferable. These processes must in turn be accessible to all concerned, from the support worker working towards a qualification structure, to the nursing student who is building a portfolio of evidence for his or her preregistration outcomes. It could be argued that the preregistration outcomes and competencies need to match, or at least correspond to, units of competence contained within S/NVQ awards at both levels 2 and 3 in Care. This correlation will be looked at in depth in Chapters 4 and 5.

In common with the other national strategic documents, *Caring for Scotland* also raises the issues of recruitment and retention of all staff. It calls for the development of a methodology tool that will enable strategic, responsive workforce planning, and the need for good staff retention records. It also makes recommendations that the bigger picture of workforce planning must inform nursing student intake.

In line with the context of this book, the Scottish strategy recommends that you consider the resource implications for nurses when assessing, delegating and supervising the work of nursing students and support workers.

CONCLUSION

Scotland is seen to be proud of its nursing education, and one of the continued aims is to develop students with the technical, personal and caring knowledge and skills required of a registered nurse. This reflects the need for competence, and reflects key words contained within the definitions of competence in Chapter 3.

The document concurs with the other publications discussed in this chapter in respect of widening the entry gate to preregistration programmes, and recommends action for education providers, within the NMC frameworks and rules, along with the Scottish Credit and Qualifications Forum (SCQF). It raises the issue of exploiting Assessment of Prior (Experiential) Learning (AP(E)L), and other processes, such as open learning, to widen entry gates further into, and through, nursing programmes.

The Scottish recommendations on the award of academic qualifications are less absolute than the Welsh, suggesting that students can work to either diploma or degree level within the same programme, and that education providers will aim for an 80% graduate output at the point of registration by 2005. Both these recommendations however give definite time scales for implementation, unlike the English strategy which suggests that targets will be achieved over an unspecified period of time.

REFERENCES

Department of Health (DoH) 1999a Making a difference: strengthening nursing, midwifery and health visiting contribution to health and healthcare. DoH, London

Department of Health (DoH) 1999b Agenda for change: modernising the NHS pay system. DoH, London

Department of Health and Social Security (DHSS) 1998 Valuing diversity: a way forward for nursing, midwifery and health visiting. DHSS, Belfast

National Assembly for Wales (NAW) 1999 Realising the potential: a strategic framework for nursing, midwifery and health visiting in Wales into the 21st century. NAW, Cardiff

National Assembly for Wales (NAW) 2000 Briefing paper 1. Creating the potential: a plan for education. NAW, Cardiff

Nursing and Midwifery Council (NMC) 2002 Code of professional conduct. NMC, London

Scottish Executive Health Department (SEHD) 2000 Our national health: a plan for action, a plan for change. SEHD, December 2000

Scottish Executive Health Department (SEHD) 2001 Caring for Scotland: the strategy for nursing and midwifery in Scotland. SEHD, Edinburgh

Scottish Office Department of Health (SODoH) 1997 Designed to care: renewing the National Health Service in Scotland. The Stationery Office, Edinburgh

Scottish Office Department of Health (SODoH) 1999 Towards a healthier Scotland. The Stationery Office

United Kingdom Central Council for Nursing, Midwifery and Health Visiting (UKCC) 1992a Code of professional conduct for nurses, midwives and health visitors. UKCC, London

United Kingdom Central Council for Nursing, Midwifery and Health Visiting (UKCC) 1992b Scope of professional practice. UKCC, London

United Kingdom Central Council for Nursing, Midwifery and Health Visiting (UKCC) 1999 Fitness for practice: the UKCC Commission for Nursing and Midwifery Education. UKCC, London

World Health Oraganization (WHO) 2002 Strategy for Nurse Education. World Health Oraganization, Geneva.

2

The move to a competency based curriculum: 'Fitness for practice'

INTRODUCTION

As outlined in Chapter 1, the nursing and midwifery strategies of the four countries of the UK were aimed at modernising the National Health Service in order to make the provision of care more responsive to changes in patient need. The development of the strategies coincided with a review of the way preregistration programmes were structured to meet these changing needs and this work was initiated and led by the UKCC, the statutory body responsible for the governance of nurses, midwives and health visitors at that time. (The UKCC was replaced by the NMC on 1 April 2002; see Ch. 1 and Glossary.)

The purpose of this chapter is to overview the work undertaken by the UKCC that led to increased emphasis on the importance of the practical nature of nursing. This also led to recognition of the need to develop systems capable of identifying, teaching and assessing the competencies required to provide high levels of patient/client care.

STATUTORY RESPONSIBILITIES

One of the statutory responsibilities of the UKCC was to set standards for pre-registration nursing education. Their last review in 1986 (UKCC 1986) led to the development of new preregistration programmes under the common title of Project 2000. Throughout 1996 and 1997, the Nursing and Community Health Care Nursing, Midwifery and Joint Education Committees of the UKCC examined and evaluated the effectiveness of the preregistration curricula, leading to the invitation of Sir Len Peach to chair their Commission for Education, starting in 1998. The remit of the Commission was 'to prepare a way forward for preregistration nursing and midwifery education that enables fitness for practice based on health care need.'

LEARNING OBJECTIVES

After reading this chapter you should be able to:

◆ review the UKCC Education Commission document *Fitness for practice* (UKCC 1999a), and evaluate the implementation of the recommendations to date

◆ understand the outcomes and competencies developed for the preregistration curricula, implemented from September 2000

◆ review the impact of EU legislation and their impact upon developments within the UK

◆ understand the development and function of the new Nursing and Midwifery Council

◆ understand the validation processes applied by the Quality Assurance Agency (QAA)

◆ understand the role of the Qualifications and Curriculum Authority (QCA) and the Scottish Qualifications Authority (SQA)

Whereas the nursing strategies are specific to the four countries of the UK, the UKCC commission, chaired by Sir Len Peach, led to the production of recommendations, which apply to all preregistration nursing programmes across all four countries. These recommendations ultimately led to the development of an outcomes and competence based framework for preregistration nursing education programmes and new assessment strategies linked to this framework.

FITNESS FOR PRACTICE

As stated in the introduction to this chapter, the commission was asked to 'prepare a way forward for preregistration nursing and midwifery education, that enables fitness for practice based on health care need.' (UKCC 1999a, p. 2). The consultation exercise was extensive, ranging from verbal and written submissions from individuals and organisations, through to focus groups. As a result, a large amount of evidence was collected which informed the material and recommendations later contained within the commission's document.

At the end of the consultation period, despite the different sources of evidence, and the varied roles and involvement in preregistration education for nurses and midwives, consensus was evident in a number of areas, to be identified later in this chapter.

The report noted that there was a decline in the numbers of newly qualified nurses and midwives registering between the periods 1993–4 and 1997–8. The Government has subsequently reviewed the numbers of registered nurses working in the UK, and identified that greater numbers needed to enter preregistration nursing programmes in order to increase the numbers of registered nurses working in the NHS. This has now occurred. However, in the interim period, the increased numbers of nursing students and the concomitant low number of qualified support staff is creating greater demands on practice placements, and especially on staff who need to assess nursing students against the new outcomes and competencies within the new curricula. In the short term this recruitment drive is affecting nurses who act as assessors in placement areas, but in the long term the increased numbers of registered nurses in the future should lead to a wider dissemination of assessor roles across these staff.

Within the document, the UKCC also recognised the paradox of increased need for extended technical competence, coupled with the continuing expectation that nurses and midwives will provide holistic care. Within education, holistic care can be further expanded to include the need to support students, of whatever discipline and level, which further adds to staff workload.

The research undertaken by the commission identified the concerns of employers, students and the public about the lack of practice skills nursing students had at the point of registration. The commission therefore placed a great emphasis on the need for the production of knowledgeable doers based on the integration of theory and practice. For this to occur the recommendation was to refocus preregistration education on outcomes-based competency principles.

The UKCC noted from the evidence they collected that the purchasing arrangements in relation to preregistration nursing education are different across the four countries of the UK. The need for stronger partnerships between the purchaser and the provider is recognised and expected to be developed.

Recommendations

The Commission made 33 recommendations, some for short-term implementation, and others requiring further work. An example of further work was discussion of the current branch structures within preregistration education programmes and the extent to which they would meet future patient need.

The document recognised the nursing strategies of the four UK countries (as discussed in Ch. 1), and also the changes taking place in the statutory and regulatory bodies. Both of these would have a crucial role to play in the debate around branch structures.

The recommendations fell into three areas:

1. increasing flexibility

2. achieving fitness for practice

3. working in partnership.

Increasing flexibility

The Commission recommended that career information and advice should be readily available, and that recruitment of potential nursing students should be the joint responsibility of service providers and higher education institutions (HEIs). It recommended that the work currently being undertaken to offer access courses should continue, and the use of Accreditation of Prior and Experiential Learning (AP(E)L) be introduced (see Ch. 6). Both of these measures are intended to widen the entry gate into preregistration programmes.

The Common Foundation Programme

It was recommended that the Common Foundation Programme (CFP), which comprised the first 18 months of the programme, be reduced to 1 year, with a subsequent increase in the length of the branch programme to 2 years. It was suggested that the CFP should be taught in the context of all four branches, i.e. Adult, Child, Mental Health and Learning Disability, and that all students should reach a common level of competence at the end of year 1, at the point of entry to their chosen branch. As we will see later in this chapter, the outcomes and competencies that have been developed for the preregistration programme reflect this recommendation.

Although the UKCC recognised the need to retain students throughout the 3-year programme, the evidence collected supported the notion of credit being given to students who did not complete the total programme. As a result they recommended that:

> students who choose to leave the preregistration nursing or midwifery programmes having completed at least year 1/CFP should be able to benefit from their academic and practice credit by having it mapped against other credit frameworks regulated by the statutory regulatory authorities in each of the four countries. (UKCC 1999a, p. 29)

Time will tell to what extent this recommendation is utilised.

Choice of branch

Many individuals and organisations submitting evidence to the Commission recognised that branch choice is a difficult decision for potential students to make without prior experience of those specific environments and client groups. The Commission acknowledged the need for greater flexibility within preregistration nursing programmes regarding the point at which a branch is selected, with opportunity also being given to students to change branches at the end of the CFP. Whilst this approach seems logical – we do not ask patients to make decisions without giving them the information on which to make an informed choice – in reality it is proving very difficult to implement. This is due to the fact that, in England, places and branch numbers are determined by workforce planning mechanisms linked to funding streams. This means that the required number for each of the branches is set before the start of the programme.

Finally, in contrast to the strong direction given in *Realising the potential* (NAW 1999) regarding the potential graduate status of preregistration programmes, the UKCC 'urges an expansion of graduate preparation for nursing and midwifery', therefore falling short of a definite recommendation for an all-graduate exit from the programme and entry to the profession.

Achieving fitness for practice

In this section, the report recommended that the standards required for entry to the UKCC register should be written in terms of outcomes for theory and practice, and that the 50% of the programme devoted to practice should become more 'transparent'. The Commission also identified the absolute necessity for adequate and consistent clinical supervision and support for students in a supportive learning environment during all practice placements.

The role of assessor

The Commission recommended that all those involved with the process of learning, including students and mentors/assessors, should know what is expected of them, through the use of specified practice outcomes, forming part of a formal learning contract, and giving direction to practice placements. These need to be jointly negotiated between the service providers and Higher Education Institutions (HEIs). This recommendation strengthens and clarifies roles in respect of assessment. The document goes on to say that portfolios of practice experience should be extended to demonstrate a student's fitness for practice, and provide evidence of rational decision making and clinical judgement. This highlights the need for the mentors/assessors to be the gatekeepers to high and acceptable standards of practice, which are assessed against the outcomes and competencies of the programme. This gatekeeping role is further emphasised in the document by stating that the portfolio of evidence should be assessed using rigorous practice assessment tools that clearly identify the skills students have acquired whilst at the same time identifying deficits that need to be addressed.

The previous paragraph highlights the importance of assessors within the educational framework. Potentially, it empowers work-based assessors with stronger decision making processes, and enhances their status in the development of competence.

This group of recommendations concludes that preregistration nursing programmes should be structured to integrate theory and practice, stating that 'practice placements should be designed to achieve agreed outcomes which benefit student learning and provide experience of the full 24 hour per day, and seven days per week nature of health care' (UKCC 1999a, p. 41).

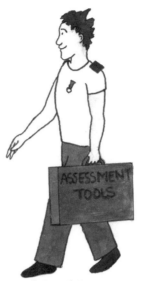

Work-Based Assessment

The 3 year programme should culminate in a period of supervised practice of at least 3 months, and it is suggested that this period of consolidation 'be managed by specifically prepared nurses and midwives' (UKCC 1999a, p. 43).

Working in partnership

The issues of partnership and ownership of preregistration education represented a large part of evidence submitted to the Commission. The recommendations identified that service providers and HEIs should support:

- their respective commitments to students
- joint awareness and development of service and education issues
- delivery of learning in practice
- defining responsibilities for underpinning learning in practice
- monitoring the quality of practice placements.

The report goes on to call for supported, dedicated time in education for practice staff, and supported, dedicated time for educators in practice, to ensure that practice staff are competent and confident in teaching and mentoring roles, and lecturers are confident and competent in the practice environment. This recommendation has major implications for employers and individuals within both settings, and, undoubtedly, there will be uncertainty and unease in some areas. It raises the whole issue of competence of both educators and service staff in areas which may at first glance seem distant from their intended roles. However, all parties need to be able to support learners within their respective environments, to enable the learner to link theory and practice, and apply both to the delivery of care.

Recommendation 28 in this section further emphasises the needs of assessors and mentors in the learning environments, and states that 'service providers and HEIs should formalise the preparation, support and feedback to mentors of preregistration students' (UKCC 1999a, p. 50). The English National Board (ENB), in conjunction with the Department of Health (DoH), subsequently published guidance relating to this (ENB & DoH 2001). This will be discussed further in Chapter 5.

THE EUROPEAN CONTEXT

It is important to note that although developments relating to nursing within the four countries of the UK are becoming increasingly devolved, all four countries must fulfil the recommendations laid down by the European Union (EU). One organisation specifically relevant to developments in nursing is the EU Advisory Committee on Training in Nursing (ACTN), which has recently recommended the specification of relevant qualifications, the minimum length of training, the ratio of theory to practice, and the content of the programmes leading to registration.

The ACTN in conjunction with the Advisory Committee for the Training in Midwifery (ACTM) (EU 1996), has demonstrated that nursing and midwifery education throughout the UK differs from that of other members of the EU in a number of respects:

- the UK is the only country in Europe which does not prepare a generalist nurse

- the current preregistration Adult Nursing Branch programme (part 12 of the UKCC/NMC register) meets the requirements of the existing EU directives, but the other three branches do not.

In reality, this means that people entered onto the parts 13, 14 and 15 of the NMC register for the Mental Health, Learning Disability and Child branches may have limited mobility and employability in other parts of Europe.

This issue is addressed in Recommendation 17 of the UKCC Education Commission for Nursing, Midwifery and Health Visiting (UKCC 1999a, p. 40) which states that 'the current programme of four branches of nursing should be reviewed in the light of the changing health care needs. The review should consider a range of options including a redefinition of branch structures and generalist nurse preparation.'

As already noted, preregistration nursing programmes will be based on defined competencies. The EU, ACTN and ACTM define competence as 'the personal attributes (knowledge, abilities and attitudes) which enable individuals to function autonomously in the workplace, to improve their performance continuously and to adapt to a rapidly changing environment' (EU 1998).

ACTIVITY 2.1	Compare this definition with others given in Chapter 3, and consider the similarities, overlaps and differences.

REQUIREMENTS FOR PREREGISTRATION NURSING PROGRAMMES

This section discusses the report *Requirements for preregistration nursing programmes* (UKCC 1999b).

Following the publication of *Fitness for practice* by the UKCC Education Commission, a working party was convened to address the issues the document raised in relation to the outcomes of preregistration nursing programmes.

The recommendations in *Fitness for practice* identified that the standards required for registration of nurses on parts 12, 13, 14 and 15 of the NMC register should:

- be constructed in terms of outcomes for theory and practice
- make the 50% practice component of the course hours transparent
- require consistent clinical supervision in a supportive learning environment during all practice placements.

Students and mentors/assessors should know what is expected of them through specified practice outcomes which:

- form part of a formal learning contract
- give direction to practice placements
- are jointly negotiated between the service providers and HEIs.

Practice placement outcomes should be designed to achieve agreed outcomes, which benefit student learning and provide experience of the full 24 hour per day and seven day per week nature of health care.

In order to allow the development of the outcomes and competencies intended by the UKCC, the content of programmes was not defined by legislation in order to allow flexibility and development by HEIs. This has enabled HEIs to develop curricula in partnership with their service providers according to local need. However, this process may complicate issues for nursing students in relation to commonality and transferability of the curriculum. Additionally, one process which seems to be particularly problematic at the time of writing, is the use of Accreditation of Prior and Experiential Learning (AP(E)L). In theory, this enables individuals to access and fast track education programmes by claiming competence in a variety of areas, whether theory based (e.g. an A-level in biology), or practice based (e.g. an NVQ level 3 in Care). This issue will be discussed in Chapter 6.

The UKCC work on developing the preregistration competencies and outcomes identified that the outcomes for the end of year 1 must be achieved before progression to the selected branch programme. Similarly, the competencies have to be achieved at the end of the branch programmes before an individual may enter the appropriate part of the NMC register. By definition, the CFP is the foundation of the programme on which all further nursing preparation is based. The UKCC suggests that the CFP should involve experience for all students in each designated branch, i.e. Adult, Mental Health, Child, and Learning Disability. This is recommended so that transferability for students to different HEIs can be assured. However, this is a very difficult, if not impossible, challenge for a number of reasons. The most obvious reason is the sheer volume of numbers of students involved in programmes, which in some universities is set at around 600 students in a particular cohort. Imagine trying to put this many students through all areas in one year, when bottlenecks already exist in some areas including Child and Mental Health placements. At the time of writing, a number of universities, in partnership with service providers, are attempting to find solutions to this problem through innovative use of placements and an expanded search for appropriate placements.

A second reason for a potential shortfall in achieving this recommendation is linked to the current processes for workforce planning where numbers for each branch are determined by future needs for qualified staff in those areas. This is a complex process, which might be seen by some as a best guess scenario.

The report recommended that the content of the CFP should be extended into branch programmes with the intention of shared learning between the branches. Branch programmes are directed at specific areas of nursing practice. It is important to note that the report states 'specific' and not 'speciality'. This means that in effect, the branch programme is still a general preparation for practice albeit with a defined client/patient group. It can be argued that specialism does not start until postregistration experience takes place, usually at the individual's choice and direction. You may wish to reflect on the implications of this.

NURSING COMPETENCIES – GUIDING PRINCIPLES

The UKCC working party identified that it was inappropriate to define nursing outcomes and competencies as stand-alone documents, and that these would need to be clarified and supported by what are now known as guiding principles. The intention of these is to develop the philosophy and values underpinning the UKCC requirements for preregistration programmes and to supply the foundation for the outcomes and competencies. Overall, these principles relate to professional competence and fitness for practice, but cannot be separated from the notions of fitness for purpose and fitness for award.

Fitness for practice

The UKCC stresses the crucial nature of practice to nursing education and clarifies that this underpins the competencies and must be reflected in all preregistration nursing programmes. Ultimately such programmes must ensure that 'students are prepared to practice safely and effectively to such an extent that protection of the public is assured' (UKCC 2001, p. 5). As a mentor/assessor, this is your responsibility, because your accurate and truthful assessment of the achievement of the outcomes and competencies by nursing students will ensure that this principle becomes reality. Do not underestimate your responsibility to yourself, your students and perhaps arguably most importantly your patients/clients. Mentors/assessors are the gatekeepers of safe and competent practice.

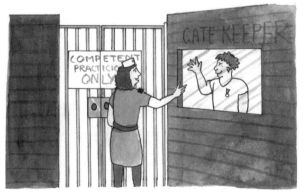

The Responsibility of the Mentor/Assessor

The UKCC suggests that the competencies have been devised to fulfil a number of functions, specifically:

- integration of theory and practice
- linkage to evidence based practice
- the use of research
- adapting practice.

Fitness for purpose

The UKCC rightly recognises that nursing must relate to the changing needs of the health service and the communities which it serves, whilst also responding to current and future needs.

Nurses must respond through their practice to the changing needs of a variety of client/patient groups. As such the document looked at a number of areas which needed to be reflected in the outcomes and competencies, namely:

- the provision and management of care
- a basis which reflects health for all
- a philosophy of life long learning
- a quality assurance mechanism linked to clinical governance.

These areas encompass such processes as accountability, delegation, and the supervision and facilitation of other workers within the health care team. This last aspect raises again the importance of your role as mentors/assessors of health care assistants (HCAs) and nursing students, to name only two groups.

The aim of all nurses, and nursing as a profession, is to achieve a high quality of health care. It can be argued therefore that your accurate and truthful assessment of competence acts as a quality assurance mechanism.

Fitness for award

The UKCC recognises within its report that 'the level of learning must be such as to facilitate the achievement of knowledge, understanding and skill acquisition' (UKCC 2001, p. 7) and within the professional scenario, this must also take account of critical thinking, problem solving and reflective capacities. The UKCC has therefore set the academic level of preregistration nursing programmes at diploma level in higher education. As discussed in

Chapter 1, within the UK and especially within Wales and Scotland, we are seeing a move towards an all-graduate exit level from preregistration programmes. England has set no time scale for this target, which always provokes lively debate.

Nursing education, alongside service provision, is faced with the dilemma of widening the entry gate whilst at the same time increasing the academic level of achievement. Much debate has centred on the level of achievement related to practice.

ACTIVITY 2.2   Consider whether the delivery of care or nursing practice improves if nurses are studying at diploma or degree level.

Fitness for professional standing

The nursing profession is charged with a responsibility to the public, and this obligation includes 'the responsibility to provide competent, safe and effective care' (UKCC 2001, p. 8). Here, the word competent appears again, and competence needs to be assessed. A number of publications are specific to nurses, including the Nursing and Midwifery Council *Code of professional conduct* (NMC 2002). Attempts are being made, usually at local level, to devise similar codes for health care assistants, and an example of this is given in Chapter 4, on the assessment of S/NVQs.

The *Code of professional conduct* (NMC 2002) reminds nurses of their accountability, both personal and professional, and implicit within this is the delegation of care to other people. Again, this raises the issue of competence, both on the part of the registered nurse when assessing the needs of patients and clients, but also when assessing competence in co-workers.

DOMAINS OF OUTCOMES AND COMPETENCIES

In its report, the UKCC divided the outcomes to be achieved before entry to the branch programme, and the competencies to be achieved before entry to the register, into four domains. These are as follows:

1. professional and ethical practice

2. care delivery

3. care management

4. personal and professional development.

The intention is that the themes develop throughout the 3 year programme, ultimately leading to a practitioner who is fit for purpose, fit for practice and fit for award.

Although the outcomes and competencies are quite detailed, it is proposed that every institution delivering preregistration nursing programmes should incorporate them into its own individual curriculum. This has caused some debate as to whether there should be a national curriculum to overcome some of the inequalities and differences identified in previous programmes. It is also argued by a number of parties that individuality leads to problems when the process of AP(E)L is needed (see Ch. 6), or when nursing students need to move to a different university at some stage within their programme. You may wish to discuss this and other issues and reflect upon how this may affect your role as an assessor with preregistration nursing students.

The Nursing and Midwifery Council

The Government NHS plan (DoH 2000) sets out a ten-year vision for nursing to take centre stage in the NHS of the future. Within these changes a major shake-up of the regulatory processes delivered by the UKCC and National Boards was announced, as well as a review of the arrangements needed for health care assistants.

The outcome in respect of regulation was the formation of a new Nursing and Midwifery Council (NMC) to replace the UKCC, and the closure of the four National Boards as part of that structure.

These changes started to take effect from May 2001, with the development and selection of the new shadow Council, to work alongside the existing UKCC. The complete handover took place in April 2002.

The UKCC was required to undergo an external review every five years and the most recent of these was led by JM Consulting in 1998. A major consultation exercise was carried out across the nursing and midwifery professions leading to significant recommendations concerning professional regulation being made to the Government in March 1999. The Government accepted most of the recommendations.

The new Nursing and Midwifery Council therefore needed to reflect the NHS Plan recommendations for the redevelopment of all regulatory bodies, which stated that they must:

- be smaller, with much greater patient and public representation

- have faster and more transparent procedures

- develop meaningful accountability to the public and the health service.

The membership of the UKCC Council was previously 60 people, 40 directly elected, and 20 appointed by the Secretary of State. Of these members, 52 were professionals and 8 were lay members. All nurses and midwives on the UKCC register (around 650,000) were eligible to vote for the 40 members. The directly elected members covered all parts of the UK and each of the four countries elected 7 nurses, 2 midwives and 1 health visitor.

The new structure of the NMC, in line with the recommendations, is smaller than its predecessor, with a total size of 23 members, 12 of whom are people on the NMC register, and 13 are lay members. In April 2001, Lord Hunt, Parliamentary Under Secretary of State for Health, announced the people who would fill the posts within the new Council, and that the structure would be:

- 1 nurse from each of the four countries

- 1 midwife from each of the four countries

- 1 health visitor from each of the four countries

- 4 lay members from an education background

- 7 lay (user) members.

The term of office for each Council member is 4 years, with a maximum of three terms in office. From April 2002, the National Boards ceased to function.

The new Nursing and Midwifery Council has written into its legislation the overarching duty to protect the public by setting and monitoring standards of training, conduct and performance for the professions. The four key functions are to:

1. keep the register of members admitted to practice

2. determine standards of education and training for admission to practice

3. provide guidance about standards of conduct and performance

4. make rules about misconduct and fitness for practice.

Although the function of the NMC is to set standards for admission to the register (including the impact this will continue to have on preregistration programmes), education following registration is not to be a mandatory matter for the Council. However, it has to approve schemes for Continuing Professional Development (CPD) for the purposes of renewal and reregistration, currently under the guise of Post Registration Education and Practice (PREP).

Many more changes will be established and implemented as the NMC develops and moves forward with a variety of agendas. As nurses, midwives and health visitors it is our individual and joint responsibility to keep up to date with and effect change as appropriate.

The Quality Assurance Agency

The Quality Assurance Agency (QAA) evaluates the standards of education provision within the Higher Education (HE) sector and within subject areas, which includes nursing. The agency does this through a system of subject review, which focuses on 6 aspects of student learning, experience and student achievement:

1. curriculum design, content and organisation

2. teaching, learning and assessment

3. student progression and achievement

4. student support and guidance

5. learning resources

6. quality management and enhancement.

Regardless of your place of employment, whether in a university or NHS Trust, the work of quality assurance is relevant to you. It impacts upon all places where nursing education is delivered, as 50% of all programmes is theory-based, often delivered within university settings, and 50% is practice-based, delivered wherever patient/client care takes place.

The Qualifications Curriculum Authority

The Qualifications Curriculum Authority (QCA) was established by the 1997 Education Act (DoEE 1997) and is accountable to the Secretary of State for Education and Skills (DfES). The QCA is a guardian of standards in education and training, and its work includes advising the Secretary of State about curricula, assessment and qualifications, as well as developing criteria for qualifications to ensure their quality and consistency, both in general education in schools and vocational training. The latter therefore has an impact upon those of you who work with National Vocational Qualifications (NVQs), as the QCA is the body that oversees their developments and uses.

The QCA does not work in isolation. Its partners are:

- The Scottish Qualifications Authority (SQA)

- Awdurdod Cymwysterau Cwricwlwm ac Asesu Cymru (ACCAC), the QCA for Wales

- The Council for Curriculum, Examinations and Assessment for Northern Ireland (CCEA)
- The University for Industry (UfI)
- The Quality Assurance Agency (QAA).

The Scottish Qualifications Authority

The Scottish Qualifications Authority (SQA) is the national body in Scotland responsible for the development, accreditation, assessment and certification of qualifications other than degrees. This body is relevant to those of you in Scotland who are involved in Scottish Vocational Qualifications (SVQs). The functions of the SQA are to:

- devise, develop and validate qualifications and keep them under review
- accredit qualifications
- approve education and training establishments as being suitable for entering people for these qualifications
- arrange for, assist in, and carry out the assessment of people taking SQA qualifications
- quality-assure education and training establishments which offer SQA qualifications
- issue certificates to candidates.

CONCLUSION

Changes in nursing education are constant and we are all affected by them, wherever our place of work and wherever we undertake roles as mentors/ assessors. The people we work with also change, as do the programmes we assess. It sometimes feels almost impossible to keep up to date with these many changes and many of us will at times feel overwhelmed and perhaps even ready to give up. We hope that you do not.

The emphasis on competency in preregistration education as outlined in this chapter means that both the delivery of nursing and midwifery education, and the structures for health care assistants in the form of S/NVQs, require experienced mentors/assessors and effectively cannot function without them. This makes mentors/assessors the linchpins for future care deliverers, whether they be nursing students or health care assistants.

In this chapter, an attempt has been made to give you an insight into the variety of work by different organisations and agencies that impact on care delivery and nursing education. There has been a tremendous amount to assimilate, and it is suggested that you use this chapter as a resource, to obtain bite size chunks of knowledge when particular situations demand insight.

REFERENCES

Department of Health (DoH) 2000 The NHS Plan July 2000. DoH, London

Department of Education and Employment (DoEE) 1997 The Education Act 1997. HMSO, London

English National Board & Department of Health (ENB & DoH) 2001 Preparation of mentors and teachers: a new framework of guidance. ENB & DoH 2001, London

European Union (EU) 1996 Nursing and midwifery education in Europe. EU XV/E/9432/7/96-EN

European Union (EU) 1998 EC WV/E/8481/4/97-EN

National Assembly of Wales (NAW) 1999 Realising the potential: a strategic framework for nursing, midwifery and health visiting in Wales in the 21st century. NAW, Cardiff

Nursing and Midwifery Council (NMC) 2002 Code of professional conduct. NHC, London

United Kingdom Central Council for Nursing, Midwifery and Health Visiting (UKCC) 1986 A new preparation for practice. UKCC, London

United Kingdom Central Council for Nursing, Midwifery and Health Visiting (UKCC) 1999a Fitness for practice: the UKCC Commission for Nursing and Midwifery Education. UKCC, London

United Kingdom Central Council for Nursing, Midwifery and Health Visiting (UKCC) 1999b Requirements for preregistration nursing programmes. UKCC, London

United Kingdom Central Council for Nursing, Midwifery and Health Visiting (UKCC) 2001 Requirements for pre-registration nursing programmes. UKCC, London

World Health Organization (WHO) 2000 Nurses and midwives for health: European strategy for nursing and midwifery education. WHO, Geneva

3

Assessment in practice

INTRODUCTION

Assessing students' competence in practice is an essential element of the role of a registered nurse and, as identified in Chapter 2, is clearly laid down in the NMC *Code of professional conduct* (NMC 2002). This means that all nurses, midwives and health visitors have a teaching element in their role. This could be either formally as a recognised mentor/assessor to a pre- or postregistration student, or an informal one that may involve providing support and guidance on a daily basis to the students with whom you come into contact. Within the context of this chapter the term student applies to any learner, from health care assistant to consultant nurse.

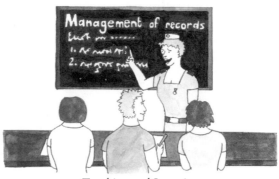

Teaching and Learning

There has been much debate about the definition of the terms mentor and assessor. Historically, the mentor was the person who provided support and guidance in practice whilst the assessor evaluated the student's competence.

Increasingly however the terms are used interchangeably: 'the term mentor is used to denote the role of the nurse, midwife or health visitor who facilitates learning and supervises and assesses students in the practice setting' (ENB & DoH 2001, p. 9).

Whilst it may be difficult to differentiate between the roles of assessor and mentor, it is equally difficult to explore assessment in isolation from the principles of learning and teaching as applied to nursing practice. The *New Lexicon Webster's Dictionary* (1991) gives the following definitions:

1. Assessment: 'to judge or decide the amount, value, quality or importance of, to evaluate'

2. Learning: 'to acquire knowledge of or skill in by study, instruction, practice or experience'

3. Teaching: 'to give instruction to, to train, to give another knowledge or skill.'

So, with this in mind, whilst this chapter's main aim is to look at the assessment of students in practice, it also outlines some of the ways in which we learn, as this is an integral part of the assessment process.

LEARNING OBJECTIVES

By the end of this chapter you should be able to

◆ discuss why robust assessment strategies are essential to high standards of patient/client care

◆ outline some appropriate models, which can be used in assessing competence to practise.

◆ identify some of the different methods of assessment used in practice

◆ recognise the value of learning contracts to the assessment process

◆ identify and discuss some of the ways in which we learn in and from practice

◆ explain some of the learning theories that underpin learning in practice

WORKPLACE LEARNING

Increasingly the workplace is seen as a valuable place in which to learn about health care. The fact is not altogether surprising as it is a place in which there is an inestimable amount of knowledge and expertise that can readily be passed on, while at the same time enabling the student to be supported by experienced individuals who are actually doing the job.

Recent government initiatives – in particular the advent of the NHS University and the education proposals in Scotland (SEHD 2001) – have placed a great deal of emphasis on work based learning not just for nurses and other health care professionals but for everyone providing health care, including, for example, portering and hotel services. As identified in the first two chapters of this book, there has been a major refocusing of nursing education

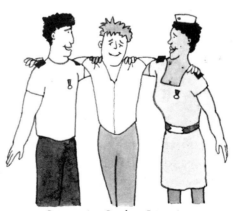

Supporting Student Learning

in practice since 2000, coupled with recognition of the need to ensure that nurses and midwives are fit for practice at the time of registration. This refocusing and reemphasis of nursing education in practice has resulted in the redefining of nurse educator roles to ensure that students effectively learn and are supported in practice. These roles are further explored in Chapter 5.

ASSESSING COMPETENCE – DEFINING TERMS

Competence is a fashionable word and appears to have different definitions depending upon who is using it, and what they are using it for! Within the plethora of available definitions, reference is made to observable behaviours including skills, and unobservable attributes, including the rather subjective issue of attitudes. Benner (1984) uses the term competence to illustrate the development of a variety of traits that enable progression from novice to expert.

Benner highlights the interface between theory and practice as applied to learning and outlines five levels of proficiency through which students progress in their learning journey: novice, advanced beginner, competent practitioner, proficient nurse and expert. It is important to note that this is not a single progression, and students can effectively move up and down the proficiency levels. An example of this would be an expert nurse in renal nursing who then decided on a career move into the care of children.

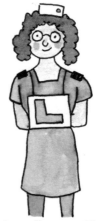

Novice to Expert to Novice

Benner identifies the novice as a new nurse who has been taught the principles of basic skills. In the novice stage, whilst being able to undertake the skill, the nurse would be unable to place it in its context or adapt it in any way.

The advanced beginner involves the student with the support of a mentor to identify the frameworks in which he/she must work. The competency stage is reached when the nurse has acquired experience in her role. Benner suggests that this stage can be greatly enhanced by the mentorship process.

The proficient nurse is able to demonstrate that he/she draws deeply on previous experiences which he/she is able to adapt appropriately to the current situation. The expert practitioner demonstrates an intuitive grasp on the situations with which he/she is faced. This involves the apparent unconscious actions in assessing planning implementing and evaluating care within a very complex environment.

Why we need to assess competence

At the root of assessing competence in nursing, midwifery and health visiting is the fact that it is a practice based profession and as such requires an agreed standard of proficiency in order to ensure patient safety. This is underpinned by the necessity for us to base our practice on evidence. Hamer and Collinson (1999, p. 6) state that 'As a process evidence based practice is about finding, appraising and applying scientific evidence to the treatment and management of health care.' It should be clear from this that if scientific evidence is to be demonstrated in the care you provide then by the same token you must have evidence of competence to practise. In short, assessing learning in many ways is not unlike ensuring your practice is evidence based, in so much as when you are assessing a student you are looking for the evidence that learning has actually taken place.

Assessing practice

Historically, assessment of nursing practice has not been seen as a fundamental part of university life:

> The assessment of practice is often uncomfortable, approximate, and problematic, but it is not an issue academics can evade, as increasingly the nature of what we assess in universities is changing from a focus on knowledge and understanding towards students' abilities to do useful things with what they have learned. (Brown 1999, p. 104)

ACTIVITY 3.1 Based on your previous experiences jot down why it is unlikely that traditional methods of assessment in higher education would effectively assess learning in practice.

You will probably have identified that assessment of theory as a rule informs us of what the student knows as opposed to what a student can do. Clearly you cannot assess what a student can do by asking them to write an essay, but you could however find out what they know from using this method. Castling (1996) sums this up neatly when she states 'you would not use a written test to judge someone's competence to pilot a plane'. In this respect nursing is no different. These issues are further explored later in this chapter.

Measuring achievement

Tallantyre (1992) identifies four areas from which evidence of achievement can be measured. These are performance evidence, product evidence, prior learning and evidence from current learning. All four of these are particularly relevant to nursing education and the assessment of students in practice.

1. Performance evidence. This relates to evidence collected from student observation in a real situation, for example the taking of blood pressure or the administration of medicines.

2. Product evidence. This requires the student to submit a product that meets the learning outcomes as set. The product could be a study and analysis of a local community or a paper for discussion at a future seminar.

3. Prior learning. This involves the need to identify the skills that students already possess and how they can be applied to the current learning situation. For example, formal education certificates (GCSE and A-level) that would demonstrate a student's understanding of information technology and its transferability to health care requirements in that field. This is also readily identifiable as students progress through their common foundation and branch programmes, gaining in experience along the way. The student as a result presents for placement with a range of skills previously learned.

4. Evidence from current related learning. This could involve learning which has been acquired as a result of working for an organisation closely linked to the health care professions – for example the Samaritans, or SCOPE. The performance and product evidence will be discussed further in Chapter 5 and prior learning and evidence from current related learning in Chapter 6.

In order to establish whether or not a student is a competent practitioner in a professional context, it is essential to use experiential approaches for the testing of skills, otherwise we risk missing the very heart of what it is that we are aiming to assess. (Brown et al 1996)

Brown et al (1996) also identify 10 key reasons as to why we should assess:

1. to clarify or grade students

2. to enable student progression

3. to guide improvement

4. to facilitate student choice of options

5. to diagnose faults and enable students to rectify mistakes

6. to give us feedback on effectiveness of teaching

7. to motivate us to learn

8. to provide statistics for the course

9. to enable grading and final degree classification

10. to add variety to students' learning experience and add direction to teaching.

ACTIVITY 3.2

In terms of assessing students in practice which of the above do you feel are the most important? Try to rank these in order of importance from the list provided.

You could rightly argue that the grading of students identified at point 1 is the most important on the list if your main interest is whether or not a student has the competence to undertake a particular skill. You may also have ranked 2 quite highly. In nursing, student progression is crucial, for example preregistration students are required to meet the outcomes of the common foundation programme before progressing into the branch. Equally, the diagnosis of fault (5) and guiding improvement (3) (in a safe environment – away from direct patient/client care) provides an effective way of enabling students to overcome any difficulties they are experiencing. Motivation (7) and teacher feedback (6) are vitally important to student learning but do not affect the fact that we must demonstrate a certain level of skill to be deemed to be fit to practise as a registered nurse.

Possibly lower down the list when applied to assessment in practice is choice of options (4). Probably somewhere in the middle of your list sits the grading and final degree. Learning in practice is increasingly being seen within higher education as legitimate learning towards an academic award.

Using models of competency

There are three main types of competence models:

1. What people are like – personal competence model

2. What people need to possess – educational competence model

3. What people need to achieve – performance outcomes/standards model.

Clearly all of these are crucial to the provision of high quality patient/client care.

PERSONAL COMPETENCE MODEL

This model relates to the personal qualities of individuals, including skills, motives and goals. These qualities impact not only on people's ability to perform, but also their motivation to do so. This model can be best utilised in personal development plans (PDPs), and for review purposes. Its use however is exceedingly limited as a means of assessing an individual's suitability for practice, as the assessment is not made against agreed benchmarks of practice or competencies. Potentially this model can be detrimental to the assessment of competence, as it tends to use a norm-referencing approach, comparing 'good' with 'bad'.

EDUCATIONAL COMPETENCE MODEL

This is perhaps more commonly referred to as aims and objectives, i.e. what someone is expected to know, or will be able to do, at the end of a period of learning, very much like the learning objectives at the beginning of this chapter. The assessment of competence based learning modules is set against agreed criteria, sometimes with a grading result involved. This model is clearly demonstrated in the leaning outcomes and competencies for pre-registration nursing programmes (UKCC 1999) and will be discussed later in this chapter. The assessment protocols within this model will identify the knowledge, understanding and skills of the specified learning outcomes. Arguably, the definition of competence which best fits this method, and incorporates the personal competence model, is that of the World Health Organization which suggests 'competence requires knowledge, appropriate attitudes, and observable mechanical and intellectual skill, which together, account for the ability to deliver a specified professional service' (WHO 1988).

PERFORMANCE OUTCOMES/STANDARDS MODEL

This model concentrates upon the outcomes which anyone who undertakes a specific role is expected to achieve. The expected levels of achievement are set by consensus and tend to focus on minimum standards of safe practice. This approach is utilised in the formation of National Occupational Standards, which are the building blocks of the Scottish and National Vocational Qualifications (S/NVQs). National Occupational Standards are devised by the relevant employment sector, so, in the case of S/NVQs in Care, these awards are developed by representatives from the field, involving people from practice including health and social care. Consensus decisions define the standards, and groups of standards are put together to form whole awards. It can be argued that the development of the outcomes and competencies by the working party headed by the UKCC identified in Chapter 2 also reflects this model.

Within the context of *Fitness for practice* (UKCC 1999), the term competence is used to describe 'the skills and ability to practise safely and effectively without the need for direct supervision'. A simple definition, or is it too simplistic? Hill (1997) suggests caution is needed when using simple statements, implying that they may leave too much unsaid, and may even contribute to the confusion around the definition of competence.

To add fuel to this suggestion, some of you may argue that the word 'knowledge' is missing from the UKCC definition. Indeed, the National Council for Vocational Qualifications suggests that NVQs are based on the skills, knowledge and understanding required for competence within a particular occupational area.

It is generally accepted that technical skills are essential for the achievement of competence, but it is also suggested that in nursing, midwifery and health visiting these skills must be underpinned by the necessary cognitive and social skills (NAW 2000). NAW (2000) identifies core competencies that are essential to enable fitness for practice. These include:

- critical thinking

- communication skills

- assessment

- commitment to continuing professional development (CPD).

The issue of competence within the framework of Scottish and National Vocational Qualifications has been debated and criticised almost since their inception in the late 1980s. It has been argued that these competence based qualifications are narrow, and 'they rely on the assessment of performance in the workplace' (Purcell 2001). It could also be argued, however, that assessment of performance in the workplace is of paramount importance in the assessment of competence in the profession of nursing. If not, why is there such an emphasis about learning in, and experience of, care delivery in a wide variety of placements? It is suggested that this process, linked with the academic rigour of preregistration programmes, gives the profession of nursing its strength and credibility, and makes it a profession worthy of that title. Perhaps it is best to leave you the reader to debate the issues around definitions at your leisure.

ACTIVITY 3.3

Try to think of some examples from your practice that you would be looking for in students and would fit the three models identified.

Personal competence models   In this category you could include the personalities of the students. Are they friendly, do they get on well with others and do they have the attributes to work well in a team?

Educational competence model   This could involve what you want the students to know, for example what to do in an emergency situation.

Performance outcomes model   In this model you could include the observation of the students' ability to undertake specific skills for example administering medicines safely.

TYPES OF ASSESSMENT

Before exploring the different types of assessment it is important to define what is meant by the term. Within the context of nursing, assessment can be defined as 'the measurement of a candidate's level of competence in theoretical and practical nursing skills' (Brooker 2001). Generally, in this book the candidate can be any learner including HCAs or registered nurses, but for the purpose of this chapter the candidate will be a student or registered nurse.

Assessment is a key component of every registered nurse's role (Hinchliff 1999) and, despite the fact that care environments support a number of learners, on the whole the principles of assessment are the same, the aspect that differs being the documentation!

Wales leads the way here in supporting assessors and learners by using an 'all Wales initiative' that involves the development of 'common' paperwork across the different universities and service providers, a lesson that other countries could learn from.

There are a number of types of assessment, some of which can be applied to the practice area, and others that only truly lend themselves to academic assessment. However student learning cannot be neatly parcelled off into practical and theoretical learning. As a mentor/assessor based in practice it is vital that you have an overview of the whole programme your student is undertaking, in order for you to see how the different parts make up the whole. You will need to be aware of the curricula that your student is working through, what learning has already been assessed, and what will be learned and assessed in the future.

ACTIVITY 3.4   Obtain a copy of your students' curricula and identify where this placement is positioned in respect of the whole programme. Identify what learning came before this allocation and what goes after.

Assessment processes

There are a number of assessment processes that you need to be aware of when assessing students. These can be grouped as follows:

1. formative assessment

2. summative assessment

3. norm referenced assessment

4. criterion referenced assessment.

FORMATIVE ASSESSMENT

This method looks at the ongoing development of skills and applied knowledge which make up to the continuous monitoring of a student's progress. It can be likened to a mock assessment where progress is assessed against specific criteria, without the ultimate outcome of pass or fail, but as a learning pathway through to summative assessment.

SUMMATIVE ASSESSMENT

This is the end stage of a learning and assessment process and experience that has a clear end result: pass, fail or refer. The process uses formative assessment decisions and other outcomes to make final declarations of achievement. For example a summative assessment will be made at the end of the CFP before a student moves on to the branch programme. There must be success at the end of the CFP, involving the achievement of the UKCC's learning outcomes as specified in their requirements for preregistration nursing programmes (UKCC 2000).

NORM-REFERENCED ASSESSMENT

This type of assessment is mentioned here simply as a warning to you as a mentor/assessor **not to use it!** Norm referencing involves comparison of like or similar entities, for example student nurses. One may be exceptional in learning and practice and may set the standard by which other students will be assessed – not necessarily a good measure!

Likewise you as a mentor/assessor might assess a student against your practice and knowledge, although it would be expected to be over and above what is needed of the student. This results in the 'halo effect' – 'she is not as good as me!' – whereas students need to be assessed against the specific outcomes and competencies contained within their curricula and learning objectives. This is known as 'criterion referenced' assessment.

CRITERION-REFERENCED ASSESSMENT

Criteria will have been developed by which the student needs to be assessed. The criteria are devised from a number of perspectives:

1. The UKCC outcomes and competencies for preregistration nursing programmes

2. The respective HEI's curricula, course content and learning outcomes

3. The individual's agreed learning objectives in specific placements, linked to their theoretical learning.

In all cases except the last example, all students will be assessed against exactly the same criteria, leading to fair, reliable, objective and measured assessment outcomes.

Assessing skills

Stoker (1994) groups skills into four categories for assessment purposes:

1. practical skills: the ability to use equipment and carry out actions

2. intellectual skills: related to knowledge and how the learner applies this; concerned with activities such as planning, identifying priorities, problem solving and decision making

3. interpersonal skills: the ability to communicate, form relationships and get on with other people

4. intrapersonal skills: concerned with the student's self-confidence, self-control and awareness of her own abilities and the effect they have on others.

Methods of assessing students in practice

ACTIVITY 3.5 Take a few moments to consider the ways in which practice can be assessed to ensure that the definition of assessment identified in the introduction is met. This may be from your own experiences as a student or as a mentor/assessor to someone else.

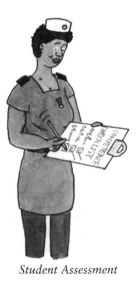

Student Assessment

Undoubtedly some of these, taken from Brown (1999), will be more familiar than others:

1. competence checklists

2. projects

3. case studies

4. logs, diaries, reflective journals, critical incident accounts

5. portfolios

6. observation

7. artefacts

8. expert witness testimonials

9. in tray exercises

10. objective structured clinical examinations (OSCEs)

11. posters and presentations

12. oral assessments

13. learning contracts.

As individuals being assessed we tend to think of the process as being absolute. For example we undertake the test and as a result either pass or fail. But how can we make sure that the assessment process in itself is effective? Murphy and Broadfoot (1995) suggest we ask some fundamental questions to ensure that it is, namely:

1. What is the assessment for?

2. When can the assessment be regarded as valid?

3. How is it possible to generalise from the results gained?

4. How do we know that the skills demonstrated during the assessment process are transferable to other situations?

5. How important is the context of the assessment. For example do students do better in assessment where they are already working as part of the team?

They also identify four issues that could potentially affect a student's performance at assessment. These are:

1. Whether or not the student is motivated to undertake the required assessment

2. The relationship between the student and the mentor/assessor. We can all identify times in our working lives when we have found it easier to relate to some staff members than to others

3. The conditions under which the assessment is being made. It is unlikely to have the best results if the assessment is to be undertaken at a time when the mentor/assessor is overworked in other areas

4. The understanding of the student as to what is required.

In addition, students perform better at assessment when the tasks that they are required to do are:

1. concrete and within the experience of the student

2. presented clearly

3. perceived as relevant to the current concerns of the student

4. not unduly threatening, something that is helped by a good relationship between the assessor and the student (Murphy & Broadfoot 1995, p. 154)

ACTIVITY 3.6 What do you think are some of the challenges in assessing students in your particular field of practice?

The fact that students are assessed practically in many different settings by many different assessors makes it extremely difficult to obtain consistency in assessor reliability. For example, how do we know that two people interpret the satisfactory acquisition of a skill in the same way? This is done by ensuring that the assessors are appropriately briefed on the assessment tools being utilised. A second factor relates to the difficulties in assessing large volumes of students with extensive portfolios when included in the assessor's day-to-day workload.

Your role in the assessment process

Castling (1996) identifies a series of questions that may be a helpful starting point to clarify your own particular role in the assessment process. These are:

1. Whose work do you assess?

2. What kind of learning do you assess?

3. Why do you assess?

4. When do you assess?

5. How do you assess?

6. Who provides the test?

7. Who recommends the level of success of candidates?

8. Who gives the candidates feedback on how they have done? (If this is a student on the ward or in the community then this is likely to be you.)

Making sure assessment is valid and reliable

There are two crucial criteria for assessment. Both are equally as important whether assessing theory or practice. They are validity and reliability. The

Little Oxford Dictionary (1989) defines valid as 'sound and well grounded'. In short this means that the test needs to do what it is meant to do. Fitness for purpose applies equally to the type of student assessment selected as it does to that of a registered nurse. Reliable is defined as 'dependable'. In short can you trust the test to give you the same result if you used it in the same conditions more than once on the same student?

ACTIVITY 3.7

Take some time to think about how you can help to ensure that the assessment process you are using is both reliable and valid.

As a practitioner, it is likely that you are involved at the implementation stage of the assessment process and as a result the criteria have already been set. It is important however that you liaise closely with the programme planners in providing them with feedback regarding your views of the process and your opinions on these important issues.

ACTIVITY 3.8

There are many different ways in which we assess students' levels of understanding and competence. Take a few minutes to make a list of those you can think of. Think back to your own learning. What kind of assessment did it involve?

Your list will include some of the following, all of which can be used in nursing and health care related studies:

- time limited written examinations
- time limited written examinations with text books permitted
- short answers
- multiple choice questions
- oral examinations
- case studies
- assignments
- quizzes
- projects
- practical performance tests such as OSCEs

- coursework
- simulation of real performance.

Ensuring assessment meets the objective

Woolhouse and Jones (2001) identify the need for the assessment being undertaken to 'fit' what is being assessed. For example, in a nursing course if you wished to assess whether a student knew the correct dosage of a drug for a child in a specific age group you could set a written test. If however you wanted to know if he/she could give the injection in a safe manner you would set a practical test – probably within a skills laboratory or safe setting – in order to assess his/her skills in actually administering the injection.

This ensures that the assessment criteria used are valid.

Questions when assessing practice

Brown et al (1996) provide us with a useful framework of questions to answer when assessing practical work:

1. What are the practical skills we wish to assess?

2. Why do we need to measure them?

3. Where is the best place to measure these skills?

4. When is the best time to measure them?

5. Who is in the best position to measure them?

6. Is it necessary to establish minimum acceptable standards?

7. How much should practical skills count for?

8. Has student self-assessment of practical skills a contribution to make?

9. Is it necessary to have a formal practical examination?

Learning contracts as an assessment tool

A learning contract is an extremely useful tool when assessing students in practice. It requires a written agreement and commitment between student and mentor/assessor regarding a particular amount of learning and the rewards and credit for the work. This has numerous benefits for both the student and the assessor. (Examples of learning contracts are given in Ch. 5.)

ACTIVITY 3.9 In what ways do you think a learning contact would be of benefit for both yourself and your student?

For your student it provides very clear documentation of what is to be achieved, when it has to be achieved, and in what way. As a result it enables the student to work towards achieving the objectives on an incremental basis. For you, learning contracts are very useful for recognising the different levels and abilities of students.

Knowles (1986) identifies many benefits from using learning contracts since they provide a way to deal with the wide differences often present in groups of students. They are also felt to increase the students' motivation for learning, and provide a much more individualised way of achieving the required competence. He identifies five key elements in the learning contract:

1. Identification of the knowledge, skills, attitudes and values that need to be acquired by the student. These involve the learning objectives for what is to be achieved.

2. How the objectives are to be met. For example, the learning resources and learning strategies that will be used to achieve them.

3. The date on which the objectives are to be met.

4. The evidence that will be presented to establish that they have been met.

5. How the evidence will be judged and validated.

Practically speaking, a learning contract is a very useful tool that enables the student to bring together theoretical learning with practice.

THEORIES UNDERPINNING LEARNING

The importance of both theory and practice as an integral part of learning is not a new concept.

> Those who are enamoured of practice without science are like a pilot who goes into a ship without rudder or compass and never has any certainty where he is going. Practice should always be based on a sound knowledge of theory. (Daintith & Isaacs 1989)

Domains of learning

There are some similarities between the models previously identified and the domains of learning as identified by Bloom (1972), in so far as they all identify attitudes, knowledge and skills as being key. This in itself is a very strong argument to support the view that assessment cannot be divorced from learning as identified at the beginning of this chapter. Bloom separates learning into three different domains:

1. the cognitive domain refers to the acquisition of knowledge, cognition meaning to know or perceive

2. the psychomotor domain relates to the development of skills

3. the affective domain involves the formation of attitudes.

ACTIVITY 3.10 Using the list you made in Activity 3.9, try to identify where the items would be likely to fit within Bloom's domains.

Examples could be as follows:

- cognitive domain: safety procedures

- psychomotor domain: drug administration, taking a patient's blood pressure, moving and handling

- affective domain: the student's willingness to work with others, and the importance of patient confidentiality to patient/client care.

Types of learning theory

In addition to learning styles, learning theories can often help us form a clearer picture of student learning in practice. Theories relating to learning are often divided into the four distinct areas discussed below.

HUMANIST

Humanist theory takes the view that learning results from enabling students. Implicit in this is permitting students to make their own choices and take responsibility for their own learning. This reflects the androgogical approach of some teachers with the underpinning beliefs that:

- learning occurs as a result of the student's own effort

- students and teachers believe themselves to be equal in the learning process

- learning and teaching strategies are student centred

- students accept responsibility for their own learning.

Humanist theory is probably the theory that nurses can most readily relate to.

BEHAVIOURIST

Behaviourist theory largely stems from research with animals which demonstrated that they could be made to respond to an external stimulus. From this behaviourists drew the conclusion that human learning could also be promoted in this way. Included in this theory is the theory of classical conditioning, first described by Pavlov. He noted that dogs salivated at the sight of food, and he termed this an unconditioned response because it was natural behaviour for the dog without any training being required. The theory is based on what is termed stimulus–response. Neobehaviourists further developed the behaviourist model and applied it much more to the way humans learn. They believed that learning should be broken down into its component parts, each being taught in a structured and sequenced way. Neobehaviourists identified the need for a reward following each component part. This could include the acknowledgement from the teacher of a 'job well done'. Woolhouse and Jones (2001) identify that early competence-based learning reflected this theory by breaking down skills into their component parts. It is quite possible that you are asking yourself how this applies to you in practice, and this scepticism is supported by Curzon (1985) who believes that human behaviour is far too complex for analogies to be made in this way. However, Nicklin and Kenworthy (2000) argue that behaviourism does have a place in nursing education when nurses are faced with a life threatening situation. Stimulus–response to the emergency is required, as opposed to conceptualisation and analysis of the factors involved.

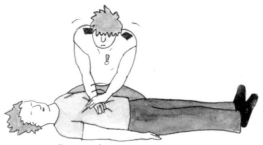

Responding to an Emergency

GESTALT

Gestalt theory identifies perception as being the key to what individuals learn. As a result much of what we learn comes from 'insight'. The belief is that once students have insight into particular situations this can then be transferred to other styles of setting.

COGNITIVIST

Cognitivist psychology places great emphasis on the individual and the belief that we all respond differently to the same stimulus. Whilst being interested in stimulus–response, it places much more emphasis on the way in which we learn how to learn rather than the learning of factual information.

Cognitivist and humanistic theories seem much more student centred, and are as a result easier to apply to our practical situation. The different sorts of learning theory are very clearly identified and discussed by Nicklin and Kenworthy (2000, pp. 46–53), using examples from practice.

Learning in and from practice

What and how we learn is obviously an essential element of the assessment process. This has often been described as being cyclical in nature (Woolhouse & Jones 2001) and is extremely relevant to education in practice. The cycle is as follows:

- identifying student needs. This may be either from the Higher Education Institution or part of a learning contract within the practice situation
- planning what the student is required to learn
- delivery of session
- assessment
- evaluation.

Individual learning styles

In practice, it is important to recognise that no two students will learn in the same way. This is because we all tend to have different learning styles. For example, some people find learning from written texts quite easy whilst others prefer visual diagram formats. Stengelhofen (1996) identifies four distinct learning styles, and places students in one of four learning categories: **activists, pragmatists, theorists** or **reflectors**. In the practice situation it may be possible to observe which category the student fits into:

- Activists are seen to enjoy working as part of a team, are open minded, anxious to learn, energetic, and easily bored.

- Pragmatists are receptive to new ideas, like things to happen quickly (need to see results) and are interested in practical consequences rather than the theory.

- Theorists are systematic in their approach to their work, analyse situations and have the ability to reason.

- Reflectors are slower to reach conclusions, preferring time to think things through before reaching a decision.

There are obviously some questions that need to be asked regarding the above model, as it makes many assumptions which could be challenged. It does however provide us with some insight as to how students learning new skills could be affected. For example, a student who is an activist may have difficulty learning when there is no interaction with others, whereas a reflector may require time to consider what is required of them.

Learning strategies

Learning in and from practice involves the adoption of strategies that help us to learn what it is we need to know, although it is likely that we do not consciously choose any one method. Minton (1997) identifies 10 of these strategies:

1. Travelling hopefully. Minton identifies this as the strategy that most people use most of the time. It is the learning that takes place on a need to know basis.

2. Indoctrination.

3. Cram it all in. This and 2 above involve rote learning often without any underpinning understanding of the concepts involved. Students frequently learn to pass exams where the memory is tested rather than knowledge and understanding of the topic.

4. Competing groups. This strategy is usually more applied to business where it is argued participants can become more motivated.

5. Interactive and group based projects. These are particularly useful in nursing allowing students to share ideas and problem solve together.

6. Tell and test. According to Minton (1997, p. 113), first you tell 'em you're going to tell 'em, then you tell 'em, then you tell 'em you 've told 'em, and then you test 'em!

7. Research and report back. This is useful where students are particularly motivated and is frequently used within continuing professional development.

8. Problem solving. Students are challenged to solve problems by critical incidents or other related issues.

9. Discovery learning. Quite literally, finding the information and knowledge as you go along. It could be argued that much of what we learn informally in nursing is acquired in this way.

10. Closed and open strategies. This relates to predictable and unpredictable outcomes of learning. For example, closed means that the outcome can be predicted, while open can change with time. When applied to the learning theories mentioned earlier, behaviourists believe that closed methods of instruction are the most effective while cognivists advocate a much more student centred approach.

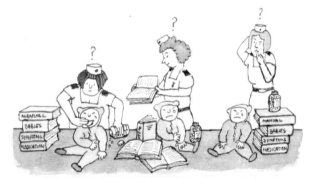

Adopting the Right Strategy

ACTIVITY 3.11 Take some time to think about your own learning and that of your students. How far do the above strategies fit into you own?

From the styles and strategies given above, it can be seen that there are many more issues in the assessment of learning than testing what the individual knows. If students are going to be given an equal chance to learn, then their differences must be considered during the lead up to the assessment process itself.

CONCLUSION

The definition of competence involves much more than learning skills. It must also involve the demonstration of knowledge and attitudes as identified in the domains discussed earlier in this chapter if nursing education is to produce nurses who are 'fit for practice'. This is clearly reflected in the definition of competence provided by Nicol and Glen (1999, p. 67):

the knowledge, skills, attitudes, energy, experience, motivation and ability to integrate theory with practice resulting in effective action to be achieved in a constantly changing, intricate and complex context.

The assessment processes are likely to be just as complex.

REFERENCES

Benner P 1984 From novice to expert. Addison Wesley, Menlo Park, CA

Bloom BS 1972 Taxonomy of educational objectives. Longman, London

Brooker C (ed) 2001 Churchill Livingstone's Dictionary of Nursing, 18th edn. Churchill Livingstone, Edinburgh

Brown S 1999 Assessment matters in higher education: choosing and using diverse approaches. Open University Press, Buckingham

Brown S, Race P, Smith B 1996 500 tips on assessment. Kogan Page, London

Castling A 1996 Competence based teaching and training. Macmillan, London

Curzon LB 1985 Teaching in further education: an outline of principles and practice, 3rd edn. Holt, Reinhart and Watson, Eastbourne

Daintith J, Isaacs A 1989 Medical quotations. Collins, London

English National Board & Department of Health (ENB & DoH) 2001 Preparation of mentors and teachers: a new framework for guidance. ENB & DoH, London

Hamer S, Collinson G, eds 1999 Achieving evidence based practice. Harcourt, London

Hill PF 1997 Assessing clinical practice for student nurses and midwives. An Aubord Itranais National Conference, Dublin

Hinchliff S, ed. 1999 The practitioner as teacher, 2nd edn. Baillière Tindall, London

Knowles M S 1986 Using learning contracts. Jossey-Bass, San Francisco, CA

Little Oxford Dictionary, 6th edn 1989 Clarendon Press, Oxford

Minton D 1997 Teaching skills in further and adult education. Macmillan, London

Murphy R, Broadfoot P 1995 Effective assessment and the improvement of education. Falmer Press, London

National Assembly for Wales (NAW) 2000 Creating the potential: a plan for education. Briefing paper 1. NAW, Cardiff

New Lexicon Webster's Dictionary of the English Language 1991 Lexicon Publications, New York

Nicklin PJ, Kenworthy N 2000 Teaching and assessing in nursing practice: an experiential approach. Baillière Tindall, London

Nicol M Glen S eds 1999 Clinical skills in nursing: the return of the practical room? Macmillan, London

Nursing and Midwifery Council (NMC) 2002 Code of professional conduct. NMC, London

Purcell J 2001 National Vocational Qualifications and competence based assessment for technicians: from sound principles to dogma. Education and Training 43(1):30–9

Scottish Executive Health Department 2001 Caring for Scotland: the strategy for nursing and midwifery in Scotland. SEHD, Edinburgh

Stengelhofen J 1996 Teaching students in clinical settings. Chapman & Hall, London

Stoker D 1994 Teaching and learning in practice. Nursing Times 90(13):1–8

Tallantyre F 1992 Portfolios as assessment tools within higher education. Morcet, Newcastle upon Tyne

United Kingdom Central Council for Nursing, Midwifery and Health Visiting (UKCC) 1999 Fitness for practice: the UKCC

Commission for Nursing and Midwifery Education. UKCC, London

Woolhouse M, Jones T (2001) Using diverse approaches. Open University Press, Buckingham

World Health Organization (WHO) 1988 Learning to work together for health. Report of a WHO study group on multiprofessional education for health personnel: a team approach. WHO, Switzerland

FURTHER READING

Nicklin PJ, Kenworthy N 2000 Teaching and assessing in nursing practice: an experiential approach. Baillière Tindall, London. Useful and comprehensive information on the interrelationship between learning teaching and assessment.

4 Assessment: Scottish and National Vocational Qualifications and National Occupational Standards

INTRODUCTION

Scottish and National Vocational Qualifications (S/NVQs) in the areas of Health and Social Care were first developed in the late 1980s to educate, train and develop the nonprofessional workforce employed within these sectors. Initially, the bodies concerned with their development and uptake were the Care Sector Consortium (CSC) and the National Council for Vocational Qualifications (NCVQ). From 1998 these changed and the bodies that then became responsible for setting standards and developing awards in these sectors were Healthwork UK (HWUK); the National Training Organisation for Health (NTO); and the Training Organisation for Personal Social Services (TOPSS). At the end of March 2002, these bodies again changed due to Government recommendations, and in the case of Healthwork UK became known as Skills for Health, which in early 2003 was officially recognised as the Sector Skills Council (SSC) for the health sector.

S/NVQs are qualifications developed by a sector for a sector, e.g. the vast health care system includes and involves public, private and independent stakeholders.

LEARNING OBJECTIVES

After reading this chapter you should be able to:

◆ understand the S/NVQ framework

◆ define the S/NVQ levels and apply them to individual roles

◆ understand the quality assurance mechanisms and processes for S/NVQs

◆ understand the assessor preparation involved

◆ apply the principles of assessment to the process.

THE S/NVQ FRAMEWORK

The S/NVQ framework provides an overarching, readily understood, and transparent national system across different levels of achievement. It also makes explicit the opportunities for progression and transfer between both qualifications and areas of competence (QCA 1997a).

S/NVQs are awarded at 5 different levels. The level descriptors are intended to be indicative rather than prescriptive, and it should be noted that the levels apply to the qualification as a whole and not to the individual units within a qualification. Not all levels apply to each sector. For example, the care sector awards cover levels 2, 3 and 4, while management awards cover levels 3, 4 and 5. Employers find the definitions of the levels useful in clarifying the status and developmental needs of individuals undertaking awards, especially those in employment.

- Level 1   Competence which involves the application of knowledge in the performance of a range of varied work activities, most of which may be routine and predictable.

- Level 2   Competence which involves the application of knowledge in a significant range of varied work activities performed in a variety of contexts. Some of the activities are complex or nonroutine, and there is some individual responsibility or autonomy. Collaboration with others, perhaps through membership of a work group or team, may often be a requirement.

- Level 3   Competence which involves the application of knowledge in a broad range of work activities performed in a wide variety of contexts, most of which are complex and nonroutine. There is considerable responsibility and autonomy, and control of others is often required.

- Level 4   Competence which involves the application of knowledge in a broad range of complex, technical or professional activities performed in a wide variety of contexts and with a substantial degree of personal responsibility and autonomy. Responsibility for the work of others and the allocation of resources is often present.

- Level 5   Competence which involves the application of a significant range of fundamental principles across a wide and often unpredictable variety of contexts. Very substantial personal autonomy and often significant responsibility for the work of others and for the allocation of substantial resources feature strongly, as do personal accountabilities for analysis and diagnosis, design, planning, execution and evaluation (QCA 1997a).

ACTIVITY 4.1	Think about health care assistants (HCAs) you work with; where would you say their role fits in the above definitions?

On the whole HCAs tend to fit either the level 2 of level 3 definitions in most health care settings.

NATIONAL OCCUPATIONAL STANDARDS

S/NVQs are based upon national standards of performance which are independent of the method of delivery, the place and duration of learning, and are detailed in the form of standards set by the appropriate standard setting body (SSB)(QCA 1997a). The standards for each S/NVQ are set out in the form of a statement of competence, which is made up of a number of units. These units of competence are known as National Occupational Standards (NOSs) and they are the building blocks of S/NVQs.

Within each unit detailed descriptions of the standards are outlined as follows:

- unit title

- elements of competence

- performance criteria

BOX 4.1	*National Occupational Standards (NOSs), Care level 2*

Unit title: Enable clients to maintain their personal hygiene and appearance (CGA 1999)

Elements of competence

- Enable clients to maintain their personal cleanliness
- Support clients in personal grooming and dressing.

Performance criteria (examples)

- The degree of support required and the *type* of personal hygiene care to be carried out is agreed with the client and they are encouraged to be as self-managing as possible.
- Clients are encouraged to use any prescribed accessories and creams which are consistent with the plan of care.

Range statements (example)

Type of personal care:

- bathing, showering and washing all parts of the body which require attention, washing hair
- shaving and the removal of surplus hair
- nail care
- oral hygiene.

Knowledge specification (example)

1. Basic anatomy and hygiene – the parts of the body which may need particular attention and the reasons for this
2. Factors which affect clients' ability to maintain their personal cleanliness.

- range statements (identified as underlined words within performance criteria)

- knowledge specification.

An example of the requirements in a single unit is shown in Box 4.1.

AWARDS

There are a number of S/NVQs and clusters of National Occupational Standards (NOSs) which can be used within and across the health sector, encompassing a wide variety of staff. For example, registered nurses and midwives may undertake management awards at levels 3, 4 and 5; and registered nurses and midwives may use the NOS in health promotion. Assessors across and within a variety of disciplines may work towards and achieve the S/NVQ assessor and verifier awards (A and V units), which are discrete NOSs from a larger award within the Learning and Development suite of awards.

The care awards at levels 2, 3 and 4 cover a vast range of staff, from care assistants working in residential and nursing homes and acute care environments, to care assistants working with district nurses, midwives and within GP practices. Managers within residential homes for example will work towards and achieve the Residential Managers award at level 4. More qualifications may be gained due to the impact of legislation, for example the Care Standards Act, which has major implications for such care environments from April 2002.

To sum up, the awards and qualifications you may meet in your work are:

- Management S/NVQs: levels 3, 4 and 5

- Health promotion: NOSs

- Learning and development: NOSs and awards at levels 3, 4 and 5

- Care S/NVQs, namely:

  - Care levels 2, 3 and 4

  - Promoting Independence: level 3

  - Caring for Children and Young People: level 3

  - Diagnostic and Therapeutic Support: level 3

  - Dialysis Support: level 3.

QUALIFICATIONS AND CURRICULUM AUTHORITY

The overarching regulatory body which is ultimately responsible for NVQs in England, Wales and Northern Ireland is the Qualifications and Curriculum Authority (QCA) and its sister organisations in Wales and Northern Ireland. This role is undertaken by the Scottish Qualifications Authority (SQA) in Scotland.

The QCA came into being on 1 October 1997. The Education Act 1997 gave QCA a 'core remit to promote quality and coherence in education and training' (QCA 1997a). At the heart of QCA's work is the establishment of a coherent national framework of qualifications, of which occupational standards are just one strand, which also includes General Certificates of Secondary Education (GCSEs), A-levels and Vocational A-levels (previously GNVQs), higher national certificates (HNCs) and higher national diplomas (HNDs).

Within the context of this chapter, the emphasis will be laid upon NVQs that set standards of performance established for specific occupations. NVQs are work based and are designed to provide open access to assessment and facilitate lifelong learning for people in employment (QCA 1997a). The Department of Health document *Working together – learning together* (DoH 2001) outlines the core knowledge and skills that all staff within the NHS should have. They are to:

- fully understand and respect the rights and feelings of patients and their families, seeking out and addressing their needs;

- communicate effectively with patients, their families and carers and with colleagues;

- value information about and for patients, as a privileged resource, sharing and using this appropriately, according to the discretion and consent allowed by the patient and by means of the most effective technology;

- understand and demonstrate how the NHS, and their local organisation, works;

- work effectively in teams, appreciating the roles of other staff and agencies involved in the care of patients;

- demonstrate a commitment to keeping their skills and competencies up-to-date – including the use of new approaches to learning and using information; and supporting the learning and development of others;

- recognise and demonstrate their responsibilities for maintaining health and safety for patients and colleagues in all care settings.

The document suggests that these core elements can be applied at different levels, for example within induction programmes, for staff undertaking NVQs, units of which can be easily matched against these core skills and knowledge, and at postprofessional qualification level.

The role of QCA therefore is to:

- accredit qualifications put forward by awarding bodies, if they meet the published criteria
- ensure the quality of the overall qualification system through working with awarding bodies
- monitor the performance and effectiveness of the awarding bodies through quality audits.

STANDARD SETTING BODIES

National Training Organisations (NTOs) were developed in 1998 to ensure that competence based qualifications are relevant to employment. Approved NTOs cover all major occupational sectors and approval is from the Department for Education and Skills (DfES). These bodies were replaced by Sector Skills Councils (SSCs) in early 2003.

Within Health, the NTO was known as Healthwork UK, whilst the Social Care sector was represented by TOPSS – the Training Organisation for Personal Social Services. These two NTOs worked closely together, often sharing key projects, such as the review of the care awards which are used across both sectors. The most recent review of the care awards began in October 2001 and will lead to new NOS and S/NVQs in Health and Social Care.

The role of the NTOs was to define National Occupational Standards (NOSs), ensure they were kept up-to-date, and ensure employer involvement in their development and assessment. Their successor bodies – SSCs – have a similar remit, but in the case of Health cover the whole of the sector, including such developments as NOSs and qualifications for porters, laboratory staff and catering assistants.

Development of S/NVQs

There are seven stages in the development of an S/NVQ:

- The establishment of the Standard Setting Body (SSB) in the form of Sector Skills Councils(SSCs).

- The SSB draws up the standards of competence which will form the S/NVQ, ensuring appropriate usage and consultation with employers.

- Awarding bodies, e.g. City and Guilds and Edexcel, work with the SSB to develop candidate assessment and quality assurance in order to ensure that the proposed standards can be delivered as a qualification.

- QCA and/or SQA considers the proposals against their criteria.

- Contracts are agreed with QCA/SQA and awarding bodies for the NVQ to be made available to the public and to be entered on to the S/NVQ database.

- Accreditation is given for a period of time, no greater than 5 years, and during this time QCA/SQA monitor the actions of the awarding body in respect of the approved S/NVQ.

- The SSB continually reviews the standards and the S/NVQ structure to ensure it remains up to date.

At the end of the agreed time period, awarding bodies make a submission to QCA/SQA for reaccreditation of the S/NVQ and potentially the cycle starts again.

AWARDING BODIES

The awarding bodies are the organisations approved by QCA to award qualifications in England, Wales and Northern Ireland. SQA fulfils both the regulatory function and the awarding body function in Scotland.

Many S/NVQs apply to, and are used in, Health and Social Care environments. As noted earlier in this chapter, the most common are the suite of Care awards, Management awards and Learning and Development awards.

The role of the awarding bodies is to:

- ensure the quality and consistency of assessment for qualifications nationally;

- produce guidance for centres approved to offer the awards;

- appoint, support and develop external verifiers, allocate them to centres and monitor their work;

- approve and monitor centres against the approved centre criteria;

- collect information from centres to inform national decisions about qualification delivery;

- provide information to QCA/SQA.

There are a number of awarding bodies offering NVQs, but in the Care framework the two most important bodies are:

- the City and Guilds of London Institute, the Care section in this body being known as City and Guilds Affinity, capturing 80% of the centres; and

- the partnership between BTEC and the Institute for Health Care Delivery (IHCD) known as Edexcel.

These bodies also function in Scotland, as does the SQA in its awarding body role.

APPROVED CENTRES

These are organisations which are approved by awarding bodies to assess and verify qualifications. Their role is to:

- manage assessment and verification on a day-to-day basis

- have effective assessment practices and internal verification procedures

- meet awarding body requirements for qualification delivery

- have sufficient competent assessors and internal verifiers with enough time and authority to carry out their roles effectively.

Approved centres come in many guises in the health care sector, ranging from an individual hospital, (often a Training and Development Department), a consortium of nursing homes working together in partnership to offer awards, or an independent training agency offering awards across a vast spectrum of qualifications. Whatever the make up of the approved centre they all have to meet the criteria stated above, though they will meet the criteria in different ways and through different processes.

Awarding bodies set criteria by which they evaluate the applications for centre approval and carry out ongoing monitoring of centres through their external verifier processes. The criteria are devised in order to ensure that a centre is:

- able to deliver the assessment process

- able to assure the quality of assessment.

Subsequently these criteria:

- help to ensure consistency in centre approval and monitoring across qualifications and awarding bodies

- specify the systems, resources and quality assurance arrangements that a centre needs to establish and maintain

- act as performance indicators against which a centre's performance can be evaluated and monitored

- establish a framework and reporting structure for discussions after approval between the centre and QCA quality audit staff (QCA 1997b).

Centre approval process

Awarding bodies must ensure that centres seeking approval:

- are clear about the procedures for approval, registration and certification

- understand their role and responsibilities in the assessment and quality assurance of qualifications.

Application for approved status may differ from centre to centre, but on the whole will concentrate on:

- an expression of interest

- advice and information given by the awarding body

- a period of development for the organisation

- submission to the awarding body

- evaluation of and a decision on the submission.

The initial approval of a centre must always include a site visit in order to approve and verify the submission and to assess the amount of further development needed. Thus an action plan will be developed with the awarding body addressing any weaknesses and deficiencies. Developments and improvement will then be monitored by the allocated external verifier.

The use of common criteria for approval should lead to:

- standardisation of documentation across awarding bodies

- consistent standards being applied across centres

- the mutual recognition of approval decisions between awarding bodies.

ASSESSMENT AND VERIFICATION IN THE S/NVQ SYSTEM

Assessment of S/NVQs has to meet certain criteria, namely validity and reliability as identified in Chapter 3. This is to ensure that performance against the national standard can be achieved in the workplace. Assessment of S/NVQs therefore involves judging evidence of an individual candidate's achievement against the outcomes and competencies outlined in the NOSs.

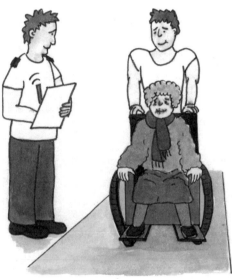

Direct Observation

Assessment of evidence, including direct observation of the candidate in actual work roles, should entail the use of a continuous assessment strategy, where the assessor takes each and every opportunity to assess the evidence and competence of their candidate. Although the assessment of practice within health care settings tends not to pose too many problems, the assessment of the knowledge specifications is different, requiring different skills from both the assessor and the candidate. However, knowledge can be implied through actions, and an experienced assessor will be able to ascertain the knowledge of the candidate through the assessment of skills contained within the performance criteria. This will be covered in more detail later in this chapter when the preparation of assessors is discussed.

Within the S/NVQ systems there is an inbuilt quality assurance mechanism, of internal and external verification processes.

PERSONNEL INVOLVED THROUGHOUT THE AWARD

The S/NVQ structures and delivery depend upon the following categories of staff fulfilling a variety of functions.

CANDIDATES

These are the people who will undertake a programme of development, learning and assessment, through which they will gain their relevant awards and qualifications. It must be stressed that S/NVQs are *not* courses, but they do entail the attainment and application of a wide knowledge base pertinent to the award. The approved assessment centre may organise off-the-job training and educational input, but the bottom line in relation to S/NVQs is the assessment of how individual candidates apply their extensive knowledge base to real job roles and work situations. This is seen by many as the advantage that S/NVQs have over purely academic qualifications.

There is no prescribed time limit to the attainment of competence (see Ch. 3 for definitions) laid down by the awarding bodies or QCA/SQA. In fact the opposite is true in order to encourage nondiscriminatory practice across the sector. However there may be employment or funding constraints which impose time scales. Most health service managers will expect and even stipulate a time frame for achievement, especially as a quality tool and safety factor in Care awards, the concern being that not yet competent implies not yet safe to deliver care.

Candidates may be employed staff, trainees on training programmes such as nurse cadet schemes, Foundation and Advanced Modern Apprenticeships (FMAs and AMAs), voluntary workers, and people on work placements from such organisations as training agencies.

The role of the candidate is therefore to:

- show they can perform to the national standards in order to be awarded the S/NVQ, thereby demonstrating the specified knowledge, understanding and skills

- take some responsibility for the quality of evidence provided to assessors.

CODE OF CONDUCT FOR HEALTH CARE ASSISTANTS

Unlike registered nurses, HCAs are not regulated. During 2002 the NMC and central government acknowledged the need to consider the regulation of the large number of staff working to registered nurses and midwives. Within the social care sector this process has been undertaken by the General Social Care Council. Debate about this process is ongoing, but as the NMC's fundamental task is protection of the public, it appears logical to some that the NMC takes on this role and responsibility.

In the meantime, a number of individual employers have been looking at the growing reliance on the nonprofessional workforce, and some have tried to structure this group of workers by devising codes of conduct for HCAs. One such employer to do this is the Oxford Radcliffe NHS Trust. Its code of conduct is shown in Box 4.2.

BOX 4.2	*Oxford Radcliffe NHS Trust Code of Conduct*

In general terms, you are expected to act in a way that:

- protects and promotes the interests of patients
- justifies public trust and confidence, and
- maintains the good standing and reputation of the Trust.

More specifically, you have a duty to ensure that your conduct does not fall below the following standards:

- Always act under the direction and supervision of a registered practitioner.
- Carry out all activities safely, effectively and to the best of your abilities, in accordance with the policies and protocols of the Trust.
- Do not take on an activity unless you can carry it out safely and effectively.
- If you do not feel ready to take on an activity, report this to a registered practitioner and ask them to help you develop the knowledge and skills that you need.
- Work in partnership with patients and whenever possible support their rights, choice, independence and self-management.
- Protect the dignity and privacy of patients.
- Respect the individuality and diversity of patients and do not discriminate against them in any way.
- Treat information about patients as confidential; disclose this information only when patients give their permission, when you are required to do so by law or when it is justified in the public interest.
- If the care required by a patient conflicts with your moral beliefs, report this to a registered practitioner and continue to provide the necessary care until the appropriate course of action has been taken.
- Do not abuse the trust that patients place in you; always protect and promote their interests and make sure that all aspects of your relationship with them are determined solely by their health care needs.
- Do not accept gifts or favours that may influence the care that you might give or might be interpreted by others as an attempt to influence you.
- Work continuously with all members of the health care team, respect their skills and contributions, treat them fairly and do not discriminate against them in any way.

(Reproduced with kind permission of the Oxford Radcliffe NHS Trust 2002.)

ASSESSORS

In relation to the assessment of S/NVQs, assessors must be occupationally competent in the areas they intend to assess, so, for example, registered nurses may assess care assistants for the Care awards, and a health care assistant who has achieved, for example, a level 3 Care award may assess someone undertaking a level 2 Care award. This is the general rule, though close scrutiny must be made of the actual units selected to make up the award and the assessors' competence across those units.

An illustration of this concept is shown in Box 4.3. The example is of a care assistant working in an acute district general hospital on a surgical ward, undertaking a level 3 Care award, whose assessor is a registered nurse.

As can be seen from the above example, assessors have to be occupationally competent, but they also need to have undertaken preparation and assessment in relation to their competence as an assessor. The S/NVQ systems have specific assessor preparation units taken from whole Learning

BOX 4.3	*Assessment of level 3 Care*

Mandatory units:

- Promote people's equality, diversity and rights
- Promote effective communication and relationships
- Promote, monitor and maintain health, safety and security in the workplace
- Develop one's own knowledge and practice
- Contribute to the protection of individuals from abuse.

Option A Selected units:

- Prepare and maintain environments for clinical procedures
- Support clients during clinical activities
- Prepare and undertake agreed clinical activities with clients in acute care settings
- Support individuals when they are distressed
- Contribute to the management of client continence

Option B Selected units:

- Obtain venous blood samples using invasive techniques
- Support individuals and others through the process of dying.

The selection of units is based around the need to develop and ascertain these competencies with this individual, and the needs of the service in relation to patient care. None of these poses problems to the assessor except the unit involving obtaining blood samples, including venepuncture. The assessor is occupationally competent in all of the units except this one, and so it is agreed to use the skills of a member of staff from within the Haematology Department, who has the necessary competence to support this assessor and candidate through this unit. The Haematology staff use this unit to assess the competence of the hospital's phlebotomy team, and therefore a number of staff have achieved the required S/NVQ assessor awards.

and Development S/NVQs, and the assessment centre must ensure that assessors have had the necessary support needed to gain these awards. All S/NVQ assessment has to be through an assessor with the relevant awards, and if they are working towards these, then their assessment has to be channelled through and supported by a qualified assessor.

Therefore the role of assessors is to:

- judge candidates' evidence against the National Occupational Standards

- decide whether a candidate has demonstrated competence

- ensure that their assessment practice meets awarding body guidance and the S/NVQ assessor awards ('A' units, covered later in this chapter).

VERIFIERS

Verification is one aspect of the quality assurance process that relates to the day-to-day delivery of S/NVQs, as opposed to the quality assurance processes of the system as a whole.

There are two types of verification in S/NVQs:

- internal verification (IV) is an approved centre's responsibility to carry out verification within the centre

- external verification (EV) is an awarding body's responsibility for verifying that assessment in an approved centre has been carried out consistently and to national standards.

Verification ensures that assessment is valid and consistent, and this is done through monitoring and sampling assessment decisions. Rigorous internal verification processes not only ensure sound assessment practice but in turn lead to consistent and valid assessment decisions.

INTERNAL VERIFIERS

A centre may have a number of Internal Verifiers (IVs) depending upon the size of the centre and the number of candidates undertaking S/NVQs. The approved centre has the responsibility to ensure consistency across its IVs. This is ensured by the development of a transparent system of verification across awards within a centre. Sampling across assessors, candidates, units, awards and methods of assessment are also tracked, audited and documented.

Internal verifiers must demonstrate:

- competence in internal verification
- possession of a relevant occupational background
- understanding of the relevant NOS
- understanding of the systems of the awarding body
- understanding of the S/NVQ system.

The role of internal verifiers encompasses the responsibility to:

- Verify assessments by monitoring assessment practice, planning the sample to be taken, often in conjunction with a team of IVs, and sampling the assessment decisions. They ensure that assessments are in line with the national standards and awarding body requirements. The IV needs to ensure that the assessors within his/her sample recognise the responsibility of the IV for validating assessment practice and decisions, as well as providing support and guidance.

- Advise and support assessors by helping them to identify their training needs and organising or arranging training for them, providing feedback on their performance, and potentially arranging and allocating candidates for them.

- Keep accurate records of assessment and verification by ensuring that the appropriate documents are used correctly, as agreed with the external verifier. The IV needs to ensure that administrative systems and documentation are fit for purpose and meet awarding body specifications and requirements.

- Liaise with the external verifier(s) allocated to the centre, agreeing and coordinating the visit, and producing documentation and evidence, including candidate portfolios as requested and highlighted by the External Verifier.

- Manage the workload of assessors, ensuring that they are not overloaded and that the demands upon their time and expertise are congruent with their skills, abilities and time.

However, there are some roles that are *not* within the remit of the IV, namely:

- Internally verifying any work they have assessed
- Re-assessing the candidates.

Education Centre Library
Southend Hospital, Prittlewell Chase,
Westcliff-on-Sea, Essex SS0 0RY
Tel: 01702 435555 ext. 2618

WITHDRAWN
FROM STOCK

The latter seems self-evident, but needs to be mentioned because external verification processes often reveal that IVs have actually assessed the candidate again, rather than ensuring consistency and accuracy of assessors across the centre.

It is preferable that internal verification occurs throughout the assessment process, and should not be left until the candidate completes an award. Most centres develop a process which entails at least three internal verification stages of monitoring, often described as initial, middle and end verification points.

To conclude, the role of the IV is to:

- Work with assessors to ensure the quality and consistency of assessment

- Sample candidate assessments to ensure consistent assessment

- Ensure their own verification practice meets national standards (Unit V1)

- Make sure that assessment and verification records and documents are fit for purpose and meet awarding body requirements

- Ensure that requests for certificates to the awarding body are based upon assessments of consistent quality

- Provide support and guidance for the centre's assessors.

The sampling of assessment decisions and the subsequent documentation produced by the internal verifiers and the centre will inform the external verifier in respect of their own sampling strategies.

EXTERNAL VERIFIERS

The role of the External Verifier (EV) is to select the assessments to be verified, based on the information provided by the centre, and to determine which candidates and assessors will be interviewed during the visit. Convenience for the centre should not influence the choice of assessment decisions and processes to be verified on the visit.

EVs normally visit each centre twice a year. The awarding bodies have reduced the numbers of EVs in each sector so that fewer EVs visit more centres. This leads to much greater EV experience and input across a greater number of centres, thus leading to greater consistency of approach and verification.

External verifiers are appointed by awarding bodies to monitor the work of approved centres. They are the key link between centres and awarding bodies. It is preferable that EVs, like IVs, can demonstrate a relevant occupational background to facilitate the whole process of external verification. Their role is to:

- Make sure that decisions on competence are consistent across centres
- Make sure that the quality of assessment and verification meet national standards
- Sample candidate assessments and monitor assessment and verification practices in centres
- Provide feedback to centres
- Make regular visits to centres and assessment locations
- Ensure that their own verification practice meets the EV award (Unit V2).

Within and throughout these roles and processes you can therefore identify a rigorous quality assurance mechanism, making the whole process – from candidate involvement to external verification, and including centre approval and monitoring – a transparent and auditable system that is open to scrutiny and examination.

ACTIVITY 4.2 Compare if you can, the quality assurance process of S/NVQ against preregistration nursing programmes and identify the equivalent roles.

You may have answered that both programmes need to have appropriate and competetent assessors:

- IV = internal moderator – perhaps another lecturer
- EV = external moderator/examiner – usually a lecturer appointed from another university.

ASSESSOR AND VERIFIER AWARDS

Throughout most of 2001, assessor and verifier awards were reviewed by the Employment National Training Organisation (EMPNTO), the standard setting body. This work has included consultation with all areas that use the existing assessor and verifier awards, D32, 33, 34, 35 and 36. This is an immense task, obviously encompassing all employment sectors, not just health, as the awards affect every single assessor and verifier across the entire range of S/NVQs. Assessor awards are structured into the following two categories.

Unit A1: Assess candidates using a range of methods

This unit is appropriate for you if your role involves:

- assessing candidates against agreed standards of competence using a range of assessment methods
- giving feedback to your candidate on assessment decisions
- contributing to the internal verification (internal quality assurance) processes.

Within the scope of this role you may be involved with:

- developing realistic and achievable action/assessment plans with the candidate
- involving other personnel as required in the assessment process
- enabling and facilitating candidates to achieve the agreed assessment requirements
- reviewing as necessary achievement to date throughout the assessment period
- identifying learning and experience needed to achieve competence
- making and keeping records of your candidates, progress and competence
- using different types of evidence provided by the candidate to assess competence.

As can be seen from this list, the role of the assessor in this unit includes:

- action planning
- review
- feedback
- judging evidence
- contributing to the internal verification (quality assurance) process.

The methods of assessment seen as appropriate for the S/NVQ, the candidate, and assessment process include:

- observing candidates performing in the workplace, which in the care environment usually means carrying out normal care roles as part of the day-to-day work of the candidate

- asking questions of candidates either because there is a gap in implied or demonstrated evidence, or to confirm the understanding of the candidate in certain circumstances, or because it will not be possible to directly observe a situation, for example in the unit related to abuse

- using AP(E)L (see Ch. 6)

- arranging simulations for elements, performance criteria and units where naturalistic observation is not an option, such as life support, or fire procedures

- assessing the candidates' evidence, including reports of their work

- using evidence supplied from other people, including peers and witnesses.

A1.1: DEVELOP PLANS FOR ASSESSING COMPETENCE WITH CANDIDATES

This element begins the assessment planning process between you and your candidate, and it is through this process that you will ascertain your candidate's understanding of the award and the assessment process. Within this context candidates will be issued with a copy of the centre's appeals procedure, highlighting the processes and actions individuals need to take if an appeal about the assessment process is deemed necessary. When collecting evidence for this award as an assessor, you will need to give evidence of how you would handle and hopefully resolve difficulties or disputes arising during the assessment process.

As an outcome of the assessment planning the methods of assessment to be used will be identified and agreed between yourself and the candidate, bearing in mind the unit being assessed and the guidelines for assessment contained within the unit and the award.

The process for assessment may be defined by the role of the assessor, such as peripatetic or work based, but all processes must take into account cost effectiveness when assessing performance.

AP(E)L figures much more strongly in the assessment methodology of the new assessor awards, and it is incumbent on all assessors working towards or working to this unit to include the use of prior experience and evidence from the candidate, obviously ensuring key areas of currency, reliability, and validity of the evidence presented against the unit being assessed.

Part of your role as an assessor is to maintain confidentiality related to the candidate, and the client/patient involved. You also need to take into consideration any special needs the candidate may identify, perhaps permanent night duty which might limit assessment or assessor access.

Finally within the planning process you will identify and agree other personnel to be involved in the assessment process, and the timescales for review, feedback and ultimate achievement of the units or pieces of work the candidate is working to.

A1.2: JUDGE EVIDENCE AGAINST CRITERIA TO MAKE ASSESSMENT DECISIONS

This element moves the assessment process on and expects you as the assessor to begin assessing the candidate by:

- using the agreed and documented assessment methods, including evidence of prior learning (AP(E)L)

- ensuring authenticity of evidence supplied by the candidate, i.e. you must make sure that the evidence is theirs!

- making decisions about the evidence submitted and collated from other sources, including your direct observation and evidence from witnesses, ensuring that your decisions are safe, valid, fair, reliable and applied to the standards you are assessing, e.g. an S/NVQ at level 2 in care and not a pre-registration nursing programme!

- identifying, explaining and resolving any discrepancies or inconsistencies in the evidence provided

- recording all outcomes of assessment, including 'not yet competent'

- seeking advice if your candidate disagrees with your decisions.

A1.3: PROVIDE FEEDBACK AND SUPPORT TO CANDIDATES ON ASSESSMENT DECISIONS

This element implies that you give feedback to your candidate on their performance and competence, both in a formative and summative manner. This needs to be done in a way that is understood by the candidate, and which identifies further action if competence has not yet been achieved.

A1.4: CONTRIBUTE TO THE INTERNAL QUALITY ASSURANCE PROCESS

This element allows you to pass on your decisions to the next stage of the process, namely internal verification (IV). This involves the documentary processes you have used within the assessment process being tracked within the candidate's portfolio and the centre's documentation systems. Your decisions contribute to the standardisation processes from the centre's assessors.

As can be identified you will need a fairly extensive and transferrable knowledge base to demonstrate your own competence as an assessor, and to fulfil your role appropriately.

The knowledge areas will include:

- the concepts and application of validity and reliability

- the Data Protection Act

- how to make assessment of current and existing levels of competence, which includes the use of (AP(E)L)

- making decisions against National Standards

- how to encourage candidates who are lacking in confidence

- the recognition of unfair and potentially discriminatory processes in assessment.

Unit A2: Assess candidates' performance through observation

This unit is appropriate to you as an assessor if you:

- assess candidates against the agreed standards

- plan assessment

- give feedback to candidates.

This unit is subtly different from the A1 unit as it concentrates solely on observation, rather than observation and other methods of assessment.

Your observation in relation to this unit will be against the national standards and follows the agreed decisions made by the holder of the previous unit, e.g. A1, in the documented action/assessment plan.

The assessment of knowledge within S/NVQ frameworks must not be divorced from the assessment of practice, and therefore you will be able to infer the acquisition and use of knowledge by the candidate through observation or through the use of, for example, check lists.

A2.1: AGREE AND REVIEW PLANS FOR ASSESSING CANDIDATES' PERFORMANCE

Within this element it is expected that the assessor will identify the best opportunities for assessing performance, aiming to disrupt normal routine as little as possible, therefore the use of naturalistic observation is to be advocated. Your candidate needs to be aware of the assessment process and timing, and agree the proposed assessment plan, including review dates.

A2.2: ASSESS CANDIDATES' PERFORMANCE AGAINST THE AGREED STANDARDS

The candidate's needs are explicit within this element, which concentrates on the preparation of the candidate and the observation of work roles, and mentions the authenticity of the candidate's work.

A 2.3: ASSESS CANDIDATES' KNOWLEDGE AGAINST THE AGREED STANDARDS

As implied by the title of this element, assessment of knowledge is the main focus of this element and, as stated earlier, the assessment of knowledge can be done through direct observation of work roles and skills. Subsequently, any gaps you identify can be assessed using the appropriate methods according to the situation and your candidate's needs.

A2.4: MAKE AN ASSESSMENT DECISION AND PROVIDE FEEDBACK

This is the end of the assessment process, and you need to make decisions on your candidate's performance based on their assessed knowledge and skills. You need to give your candidate feedback on their overall performance. This is an easy process where success and competence have been demonstrated. It is never easy to tell someone they are not yet competent, but as you work in a health care scenario, honesty is paramount when safe and competent care delivery is based upon your decisions.

The final performance criteria in this element relate to the appeals procedure in the event that your candidate wishes to appeal against your decision. All approved assessment centres for S/NVQs must have an appeals procedure built into their system, and it is your responsibility to understand the process. All candidates must have a copy of the document, usually contained within their induction pack.

Within the whole A2 unit the knowledge evidence required means that you as the assessor will need knowledge of:

- the standards you are assessing against

- issues relating to validity and authenticity of candidate evidence

- how to use simulations appropriately

- recording decisions and moving work on to the next step

- quality assurance processes

- the need to maintain or update your own assessment knowledge.

ASSESSMENT PROCESS

Now that you have knowledge of the assessor criteria and awards for S/NVQs it is necessary to explore the process you need to adopt in order to move a candidate through assessment of a unit.

You will first of all need to identify and agree which unit you will work on, and if this is the first unit within an award that your candidate is starting it is advisable to start a unit that the candidate is comfortable with. For example, at level 2 it may be appropriate to start on one of the units involved with the activities of daily living, such as *'enable clients to maintain their personal hygiene and appearance or enable clients to access and use toilet facilities'*. This starting point helps your candidate to settle into the assessment process by using a skill that most HCAs perform regularly. It may also enable you as a new assessor to become used to assessment processes and documentation.

Initial assessment

Arrange to meet with your candidate in order to begin the process. Discuss your candidate's current experience, and then identify existing skills and knowledge. Your HCA may have been employed in her current role for a while, and though no formal assessment has been documented, the HCA may feel able to undertake certain roles. This previous learning may have been through formal learning such as health and safety seminars, manual handling programmes or food hygiene courses. Although your HCA may be able to produce certificates of attendance, attendance is all they prove. They do not demonstrate learning in isolation, but may be accepted if further evidence is collected, such as a work book completed for the topic, or a statement of assessment linked to the learning, such as formal assessment of handling skills.

Remember, a certificate of attendance demonstrates attendance even if the candidate dozed on the back row and learned nothing!

Assessment action plan

Once your initial assessment is completed and documented it then forms the basis of your whole process and progress through an award. You now need

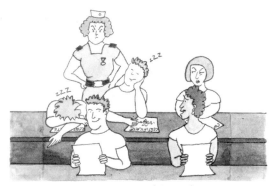

Demonstration of Attendance

to plan the assessment of a specific unit. This might sound alien if you intend to assess your candidate holistically, but a defined passage through the award is necessary because without planning, your candidate may feel she is not achieving. This does not mean that you cannot assess holistically, but rather you need to document all of your assessment of skills and knowledge, and refer the documented information to specific units as and when appropriate.

For example, you work with your candidate from 7:30 a.m. through to the end of the shift at 2:30 p.m. Throughout this time you may be working on the unit related to patient hygiene needs, but your work also includes:

- communication in a variety of ways, e.g. written, oral, nonverbal

- dealing with a potentially aggressive situation

- awareness of health and safety practices

- transferring patients from bed to chair

- documenting care delivery

- feeding patients.

All of these skills can be matched against other units of competence contained within the award that the candidate is working towards, and therefore potential evidence is generated for these units through an holistic assessment process.

Using your approved centre's documentation, discuss and document with your candidate:

- which unit(s) you will work on

- what assessment methods you will need

- what evidence your candidate needs to collect, e.g. witness statements (testimonies)

- how long the process will take – target completion date
- review dates
- how to access you!
- when you will specifically observe their performance – date, time, place
- prior learning and experience which will be taken into account (APEL)
- document (log) the agreed process and start the assessment.

When agreements have been made and documented, then assessment begins. Assessors may be employed in two ways:

1. as a permanent member of staff in the same work area as the candidate undertaking the award, such as a staff nurse on a medical ward where the HCA works

2. as a peripatetic assessor usually employed by the assessment centre whose role is to assess a number of candidates in a number of different areas, such as a registered nurse who assesses five different candidates in five different nursing homes.

ACTIVITY 4.3 Compare and contrast the two assessor approaches and identify which may work best.

Your answers might include:

Work based assessor

- always there
- holistic assessment
- can use every learning opportunity
- sees true working pattern and competence of candidate
- assessment may not be high on priority list of work to do.

Peripatetic assessor

- only arrives at agreed times
- may do holisitic assessment but may only observe identified activities

- may see high standard applied which may not be applied consistently, i.e. when the assessor is not there!

- only there to assess – no competing demands.

In the second example the peripatetic assessor needs to be constructive with her time and processes and will make appointments with her candidate and the care environment to visit the HCA and assess. This usually means a very defined assessment plan, with identified achievements to be made in the time available. This does not mean however that other evidence observed on that visit cannot be used. It is up to you to log this evidence, make the candidate aware of it, and keep it for future use and reference when the appropriate unit is being assessed and documented.

Methods of assessment

It is up to you and your candidate to decide which methods of assessment to use. Remember though that the care awards are very specific about the use of direct observation, since this is the main method for most units and elements, although there are some exceptions to this. For situations that may be rare, or unpredictable, such as fire procedures or medical emergencies, simulation may be a more appropriate method. Therefore the methods of assessment you may choose include:

- direct observation

- simulation

- questions

- projects/case studies

- evidence of prior achievements (APEL)

- product evidence.

The methods chosen will depend on the unit, the care setting and of course the candidate's needs.

Assessment centres may have and use different documentation, or may use the ones supplied by their awarding body, but it is up to you as the assessor to be aware of the correct paperwork and how to use it. You will also need to know how to pass on the evidence to the next stage of the process, i.e. into the internal verification system.

Over the agreed time you will gather evidence of your candidates' skills and knowledge as will the candidate. By the review date this evidence will be collected and collated and logged against the unit you are working with. You will begin to make decisions about the evidence based on the 5 rules of evidence:

1. Validity – does it meet the needs of the unit?

2. Authenticity – is it the candidate's work?

3. Sufficiency – is there enough evidence to infer competence?

4. Currency – is the evidence up to date and still relevant?

5. Reliability – does it accurately reflect the level of performance?

ACTIVITY 4.4   Think of items of evidence which may have a limited 'currency' value.

Your answers might include

- health and safety issues

- manual handling issues

- first aid qualifications

- food hygiene qualifications.

Sufficiency of evidence

Assessors often raise questions around the issue of sufficiency, but there is no hard and fast rule for this, rather the advice is that sufficiency of evidence will depend on the candidate's experience, both past and present, the unit being assessed, and the type of evidence produced. The only essential in relation to sufficiency is that there must be enough appropriate evidence for competence to be demonstrated, and for you as the assessor to truthfully say that the candidate is now competent, and therefore *safe* to deliver this aspect of care.

Once all of the criteria have been assessed and the underpinning knowledge base inferred directly or indirectly and assessed, then you can complete the documentation and sign off the unit, potentially passing work on to the next stage, that of internal verification.

You then move on to the next unit until the whole award is assessed and completed. Remember you may already have evidence to contribute to the other units.

Internal verification

As identified earlier in the chapter, the Internal Verifier (IV) is at the heart of quality assurance in NVQs (QCA 2001). QCA also states that the IV is a key player in managing risk, for example ensuring that when certification is claimed for a candidate it reliably marks the achievement of National Occupational Standards. This links very closely with the importance of true and accurate assessment on behalf of you as the assessor.

QCA and the health care awarding bodies identify three aspects of the IV role:

1. verifying assessment

2. developing and supporting assessors

3. managing quality of S/NVQ delivery.

Verifying assessment

Through this process the IV (remember here that you or your colleagues may have dual roles within the system: that of assessor and IV) needs to ensure consistent and reliable assessment and monitor its quality, highlighting problems, trends and the development needs of assessors. However your role as IV is *not* to second-assess the candidate!

The IV process in all centres must maintain the quality of assessment for all candidates, and therefore encompasses the work of all assessors on a sampling basis. This quality audit then incorporates sampling assessments, monitoring assessment practice and standardising assessment judgements.

Sampling assessment

Sampling means reviewing the quality of assessors' judgements at both interim and summative stages, i.e. throughout the assessment process and at the end. Interim sampling means you will potentially see unfinished work, but you can nevertheless verify the work to date in order to identify the quality of formative guidance on assessment and the effectiveness of assessment (action) planning. By using this process the IV will be able to identify problems early on and give advice and support to assessors to rectify the situation.

The summative approach will evaluate how the assessor came to the final decision, and the IV should be able to track the whole assessment process through the evidence and documentation (audit trail) and ensure that all the rules of evidence have been covered.

As assessors need to meet the requirements of the 'A' units, so the IV needs to meet the requirements of the 'V1' unit.

UNIT V1: CONDUCT INTERNAL QUALITY ASSURANCE OF THE ASSESSMENT

This unit is applicable to you if you:

- evaluate the internal assessment process
- monitor and review internal assessment audit systems
- carry out related IV or moderation activities.

The new verifier units encompass the need to ensure that health, safety and environmental protection procedures are applied within assessment arrangements, in other words the candidates are not exposed to risk when undergoing assessment. The monitoring of equal opportunities is also a requirement of this unit. In total this unit covers:

- carrying out and evaluating internal assessment and quality assurance systems
- supporting assessors
- monitoring the quality of assessors performance
- meeting external quality assurance requirements.

This latter stage moves the whole quality audit through to the external verifier process.

UNIT V2: CONDUCT EXTERNAL QUALITY ASSURANCE OF THE ASSESSMENT PROCESS

As has been stated earlier in this chapter, the external verifier (EV) is appointed by the awarding body and allocated to an assessment centre. Therefore this unit of competence is appropriate to you if you:

- externally evaluate the internal assessment process
- carry out related external verification activities.

| FIGURE 4.1 | *Quality assurance cycle in S/NVQs* |

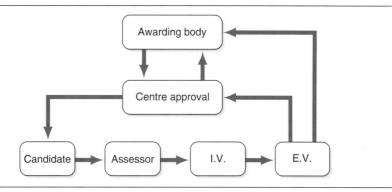

The unit and role covers:

● monitoring the internal quality assurance arrangements

● checking the quality of assessments

● providing information, advice and support on the internal quality assurance of assessment processes

● evaluating the effectiveness of external quality assurance of the assessment process.

The scope of the role is broad, but completes the quality process through which all S/NVQs are monitored and assessed and approval of centres is maintained. The direction of the whole process is shown in Figure 4.1.

CONCLUSION

Your role as an assessor for S/NVQs in Care is paramount to the delivery of high standards of patient/client care. This ranges from patients in acute hospitals on surgical, medical and renal dialysis wards, to name but a few, through to the elderly in nursing homes, and people with learning disabilities or mental health problems in community settings. Your true and accurate assessment of candidates working towards these awards goes a long way to guaranteeing safe care for these vulnerable patients and clients.

It is not a role to be undertaken lightly and must be seen in the context of the need for safe and competent care delivery by appropriate and competent staff, and, at the same time, the award of a nationally recognised award which may enable people to gain employment in many areas of the health and social care sectors.

REFERENCES

City & Guilds Affinity (CGA) 1999 NVQ in care level 2: student logbook. City & Guilds, London

Department of Health (DoH) 2001 Working together – learning together: a framework for lifelong learning for the NHS. DoH, London

Qualifications and Curriculum Authority (QCA) 1997a Vocational qualifications in England, Wales and Northern Ireland. QCA, London

Qualifications and Curriculum Authority (QCA) 1997b The awarding bodies' common accord. QCA, London

Qualifications and Curriculum Authority (QCA) 2001 Joint awarding guidance on internal verification of NVQs. QCA, London

5 Assessment: nursing programmes

INTRODUCTION

When exploring the issues around assessment it is usual to look at them in relation to the outcomes achieved by individuals as part of their practice (see Ch. 4). As a result, the responsibility for what students learn often appears to rest with those individuals who are on the 'front line' of assessment. As seen in previous chapters, assessment is a complex process that fits into a much bigger picture of health care, particularly in relation to the needs of patient/clients, employers, governing bodies, and the needs of the nurse at preregistration level and beyond. This can be divided into four key areas:

- needs as identified and presented by service users, i.e. patients and clients

- the education required by the Nursing and Midwifery Council in order for you to access the professional register and then to maintain and ensure your continuing professional development (CPD)

- the education you require as a nurse in order to meet your own goals in life, for example a job as a consultant nurse

- the education required by employers in order for nurses to do the job that they are required to do.

The purpose of this chapter therefore is to provide the context within which nurses are assessed, to identify key roles and responsibilities, and to identify how students can best be supported in practice. In the context of this chapter, the term student refers to any learner, either on preregistration programmes or undertaking continuing professional development.

LEARNING OBJECTIVES

After reading this chapter you should be able to:

- understand the principles underpinning nursing education

- identify the needs and responsibilities of employers in the education process

- understand the issues around practice placements for student nurses and their relationship to the assessment process

- identify what assessment methods are available to you

- understand and apply the key responsibilities of mentors to student support

- understand the types of assessment and apply them to the process.

NURSING EDUCATION – WHOSE BUSINESS IS IT?

When applied to nursing practice and student support, the responsibility to provide a high standard of patient/client care rests with many different agencies. It involves:

- the NHS and the independent and voluntary sectors who have a role in ensuring students are supported in practice

- the students themselves

- staff working in higher education institutions such as personal teachers, link lecturers and leaders of the education programmes

- service providers – This is taken to mean the providers of both care and the placements in which the students receive their practical experience; these will likely involve mentors/assessors and practice educators discussed later in this chapter

- the commissioning bodies for education in the four countries of the UK.

It should be readily apparent that practice education cannot be the sole responsibility of one group, as each has a vested interest in making sure that the nursing workforce is 'fit for purpose'. Collaborative partnership among everyone involved is seen as the way to make this happen.

PRACTICE PLACEMENTS

Practice experience is an essential element in most nursing programmes and as such it is vital that students are enabled to get the most from their learning experiences. As a practitioner, you are one of the key people involved in this learning and your contribution is invaluable in the context of the programme the student is undertaking. A good mentor/assessor can often make the difference between a student leaving or staying on a course when the going gets tough. You are a role model, teacher, mentor/assessor, nurse, source of information – a multi-skilled professional who can make a real difference to the student experience. That said, students are not absolved of responsibility for their own learning. This is discussed later in the chapter.

ACTIVITY 5.1   Think back to your days as a nursing student. What factors contributed to a 'good' placement?

Your list might include:

- they were expecting you!

- you were allocated a mentor/assessor

- the off duty was done in such a way as to allow you to work with your mentor/assessor

- your learning objectives were identified and met

- your mentor/assessor was keen and enthusiastic.

LEARNING IN AND FROM PRACTICE

The importance of learning in and from practice cannot be underestimated. This is stressed in *A health service for all talents: developing the NHS workforce* (DoH 2000), which identifies the Government's commitment to enlarging the health professional workforce. This in turn will lead to greater demands on professional staff to support the increase in numbers. As a result the Government accepts the need for better support and recognition for practice mentors/assessors and calls for health service managers to be more systematic in their approach to this. It is also important that there are sufficient resources, both physical and structural, available to support student learning in practice. Implicit in this is the need for students and their mentors/assessors to know what is expected of them through the use of specified learning outcomes that form the basis of a learning contract between the student and the assessor. This is part of your role, and in order to fulfill it you have to know what the student needs to learn, and then match that to your available resources. You will need to contextualise those outcomes and make them live for the students, applying them to practice within your own practice setting. ENB and DoH (2001a) suggest that in order to best support students, practice placements should:

- have a stated philosophy of care which is reflected in practice and in the curriculum aims

- reflect respect for the rights of health service users and their carers

- have an audit process which ensures that students are not placed in vulnerable situations

- enable students to experience the role of the registered nurse in a variety of contexts

- enable students to experience being part of a multi-disciplinary team.

As a mentor/assessor, you are not meant to take all of the responsibility for the student onto your own shoulders. Students are adult learners, responsible and actively involved in their own learning, and some of the onus of learning is devolved to them. However, a student will not know what they can learn if they don't know what's on offer. This is your job. You and your students need to be realistic – nobody can learn everything in one practice placement, and you will not be able to expose your students to all possible experiences.

WORKING IN PARTNERSHIP

RCN (2002) states that education and service colleagues must work together to develop innovative approaches to assessment which are valid and reliable (validity and reliability are covered in Chs 3 & 4). This reinforces the partnership approach that is vital for student support and learning, and the commitment of both HEIs and service providers to develop the learning of students. Too often it has been said that preregistration students do not belong to either the university or the hospital. Students have often felt torn between the two places, trying to fit into both, and potentially not fitting into either. You are absolutely key in supporting students in your practice area. ENB and DoH (2001a) recommend that:

- Periods of practice experience used for summative assessment should be a minimum of four weeks in length.

- There should be a named mentor/assessor to assess students in practice placements.

- This individual should have qualifications and experience commensurate with the context of care.

- The students developing competence should be assessed through agreed practice assessment strategies which identify the skills the student has acquired and any deficits that need to be addressed.

- The student should demonstrate competence through the achievement of learning outcomes in both theory and practice. (See Ch. 3: 'Definitions of competence'.)

- The use of a portfolio of practice experience should be included in the assessment of a student's fitness for practice, providing evidence of rational decision making and clinical judgement.

- The mentor/assessor should directly observe the student's achievement of intended learning outcomes for a period of sufficient length to allow valid judgements to be made. (See Ch. 3.)

Students were key contributors to the Commission into Preregistration Nursing Education (UKCC 1999), stating that longer placements were necessary in order to feel part of the team, to consolidate and begin further learning before moving to the next placement. These longer placements give you as mentor/assessor the chance to get to know your student and for the off duty to be completed to meet learning and assessing needs. Students need to know whom to approach when they arrive and who is going to support them through their placement. This again increases their feeling of belonging. A sense of belonging becomes even more important when the many different types of students that may be in the placement areas are identified.

ACTIVITY 5.2   List the types of learners in your ward/department.

Your list might include:

- S/NVQ candidates
- preregistration nursing students
- postregistration students
- medical students
- overseas nurses on adaptation programmes
- allied health professions students, e.g. physiotherapists, occupational therapists
- work experience students from schools or colleges.

PLANNING FOR INITIAL ASSESSMENT

Before anything else, you will need to undertake an initial assessment with your student, identifying achievements and gaps and areas where learning needs to be consolidated – for example, learning that has been achieved elsewhere, but which needs to be transferred to a new environment. Once you have identified these areas, you and the student in partnership need to develop a learning (assessment) contract for the whole experience, including some time for review and reflection.

PORTFOLIO DEVELOPMENT

Portfolios are a key element of learning in practice, since the student will enter their evidence into it, which in turn will serve various purposes. A portfolio can be defined as:

a personal and private collection of evidence, which demonstrates the owner's continuing and professional development. It documents the acquisition of knowledge, skills, attitudes, understanding and achievements, in recording these events. It deals with the past.

It contains reflections on current practice and progress, and in doing this it deals with the present. However, it also contains an action plan for future career and professional development, and in this it looks to the future. (Brooker 2001)

The portfolio becomes a lifelong learning document, ultimately documenting evidence throughout the nurse's career – for example through an NVQ entry route, to preregistration programmes, to a newly qualified staff nurse undertaking a period of preceptorship, through to the fulfilling of PREP CPD requirements, and onwards. Much of what you have just read will match in some ways the assessment practices for S/NVQs (Ch. 4). Indeed, ENB and DoH (2001b, p. 10) suggest that 'it will be advantageous and economic for approved institutions to develop mentor preparation programmes which also incorporate preparation for assessing students working for National Vocational Qualifications'.

KEY RESPONSIBILITIES OF MENTORS

RCN (2002) identifies key responsibilities for mentors. They need to:

- contribute to a supportive learning environment and quality learning outcome for students
- be approachable and supportive and have knowledge of how students learn best
- have knowledge and information of the student's programme of study and practice assessment tools in use throughout the UK
- be willing to share their knowledge of patient/client care
- identify specific learning opportunities that are available within the placement area
- ensure that the learning experience is a planned process
- ensure that time is identified for initial interviews with students in order to assess learning needs and develop a learning contract/logs as appropriate
- identify with students their 'core competencies and outcomes to be achieved' by the end of the placement

- make time to observe students undertaking new skills for the first time and also when practising newly learnt skills

- encourage the application of enquiry based learning and problem solving to situations rather than just giving factual information

- build into the learning experiences opportunities to experience the skills and knowledge of other specialist practitioners

- build into the daily routine adequate break times to enable students to enjoy the whole practice learning experience

- offer encouragement to students and work in partnership with the multi-disciplinary team in order to provide holistic care

- provide time for reflection, feedback and monitoring students' progress

- ensure that students have constructive positive feedback with suggestions on how they can make further improvement to promote progress

- seek evaluative feedback from students at the end of their practice placement experience

- be willing to take pride in sharing the student's journey on the path to becoming a registered nurse or midwife.

Programmes for preparing mentors

Let's consider here what a programme for preparing mentors should contain. HEIs run mentor progammes usually at academic level 3, meeting the different learning needs of mentors, students, programmes, and HEIs and regulatory bodies. The overall aim of such programmes should be to develop practitioners who actively support students and learning in practice settings, and who are themselves reflective practitioners. Contents should therefore be clustered around:

- educational theory
- use of educational theories applied to the facilitation of learning
- reflection of the facilitation of learning and assessment practice
- development of future strategies to facilitate learning and assessment in practice.

Within these four areas it needs to be identified whether the mentor student already has skills which are transferable into this learning experience. This prior learning may include reflection and problem solving, among other things.

In common with current practices across nursing programmes, the mentor student will have to collect evidence of learning, working with students in practice placements, and completing a portfolio of evidence. Along with summative assessments, this will provide the evidence of competence for the individual aiming at becoming a mentor to nursing students, at pre- and postregistration levels.

THE ASSESSMENT PROCESS

Let's now look at the way you will assess students in your workplace. In this section the following scenario will be used:

The student is a first year nursing student, half way through CFP, with successful outcomes to date. The student is undertaking the adult branch, and has previously had placements in a nursing home and a surgical ward. Your current post is working on a medical ward in the speciality of gastrointestinal pathology, caring for patients with multiple problems. The student will be spending 8 weeks with you, directly after 6 weeks acquiring new knowledge in the university.

The processes which will need to be devised, agreed and used by you and your student during this placement are:

- assessment of learning needs

- assessment of prior experience and learning (AP(E)L) (see also Ch. 6)

- objective-setting

- devising a learning contract

- methods of assessment

- feedback and reflection.

Assessment of learning needs

As previously shown, it is probable that you will have different categories of learner in your ward, including student nurses at various stages of their programme, and other learners, both professional and non-professional, such as HCAs undertaking a S/NVQ level 3 in Care. At the outset of the experience you and your student will need to identify some specific issues as a basis for all the work and outcomes over the 8 weeks. These are:

- the learning the student has achieved to date, and the need for potential consolidation of this learning

- their personal learning needs
- the learning outcomes to be achieved during the placement
- planning for future learning.

ACTIVITY 5.3   Using these bullet points and working with a student, begin to identify their learning needs. N.B. through this process you may identify learning needs of your own!

Once this has been discussed then you and your student will then be able to define and construct a learning (assessment) contact. However, before this it would be useful to mention the use of AP(E)L, though this is covered in more detail in Chapter 6.

Assessment of prior experience and learning

The notion of accreditation starts before a student enters a preregistration nursing programme. In *Fitness for practice* (UKCC 1999) there is a recommendation that the use of AP(E)L should be introduced to allow for more flexible entry to nursing programmes.

As your student is now 6 months into CFP, a considerable amount of learning will have taken place. It is appropriate therefore that at the outset of this experience you and your student discuss achievements to date, using the student's portfolio as evidence of learning, and matching this to what should be achieved in this placement. The need to consolidate that learning might be identified, as will strengths and weaknesses of the student's learning, with particular emphasis on identifying gaps which can easily and logically be filled during this experience.

For example, the student may be very capable in taking patients' blood pressure and making observations of other vital signs, but the application of the whole concept – including the theory of the anatomy and physiology of the cardiovascular system, physiology applied to the maintenance of blood pressure in health and illness, as well as the physical measurement of blood pressure including the use of a variety of technology – needs to be determined. In this learning opportunity, knowledge and skills already acquired need to be applied to a different client group, i.e. those with medical problems not requiring surgical intervention, and where accurate diagnosis of conditions may rest upon accurate measurement of such physiological events.

The outcome is that you will credit the student's competence but during this placement enable her to transfer the competence into different scenarios, with a different client group with different needs. Therefore you will have assessed and accredited prior learning and achievement.

Objective-setting

Within this concept you will need to take account of your own and the learner's needs, and the assessment and programme requirements. It is your role to integrate these areas to make an achievable outcome.

The student will need to develop new skills and knowledge, and revise and consolidate existing competence. However, before you can enable the student to move forward, the student needs to know what opportunities are available to them in your ward environment. It is no good asking the student what they want to learn if they do not know what's on offer! The learner needs to make an informed choice, but can't do that until they have been informed. Logical, you might say, but easily overlooked on busy working days.

You need to enjoy your role as a mentor otherwise you will not do it well. You need time to deliver this role, a rare and precious commodity in today's health care system, but if this is not forthcoming competent students may not qualify or may feel unsupported. Managers and others should be aware of this need and somehow build it into the process, but it is not intended to give the remedy here. You will know the learning opportunities available to your student and it is your responsibility to let the student know of them.

As shown previously, the preregistration programme will have identified and specified learning outcomes, both in the context of UKCC outcomes and competencies, and the outcomes for the curricula devised by the university at which your student is studying. Some of these outcomes will be generic, such as communication skills, and others may be more specific, such as nutritional needs of patients. You will enable the student to apply these specific outcomes when, for example, caring for patients with a percutaneous endoscopic gastrostomy feed (PEG).

Once the objectives have been identified and collated they can then be built into the learning contract.

ACTIVITY 5.4　Using your current workplace as an example, list what is on offer to meet your students' objectives.

For a surgical placement this list might include:

- the ability to observe surgery
- the ability to follow a patient through from admission to surgery and discharge
- the ability to observe and take part in various investigations
- exposure to specialist surgical procedures and investigations.

Devising a learning contract

A learning contract can be defined as a written or spoken agreement. Within the learning contract, objectives (see above) need to be agreed and documented, as this forms the basis for learning for the duration of the placement and for the future learning of the student when moving to another practice placement. The contract is not a static document but can be added to and amended as requirements change in respect of the learning that has to take place and the opportunities that may present. Richardson (1987) describes a learning contract as 'a written agreement between teacher and student which makes explicit what a learner will do to achieve specified learning outcomes.' It has also been suggested that learning contracts enable learners to develop their concept of lifelong learning (Dart & Clarke 1991). DoH (2001) suggests that lifelong learning is the process by which 'we have the right number of staff with the right skills in the right place at the right time.'

Some HEIs will have specific paperwork on which you record the learning contract, and others will not, but the contract needs to include:

- student's name

- date of commencement of the preregistration programme

- branch choice

- dates of this placement

- ward name

- mentor's name

- link/personal tutor's/practice educator's name

- AP(E)L

- UKCC outcomes

- personal objectives

- placement objectives/opportunities

- methods of assessment

- target dates – interim and final

- signatures – mentor and student.

Within your workplace, the learning contract can be used by you and the student to bring theoretical learning into the practice setting. Using the scenario provided above, as your student has just spent 6 weeks in a classroom setting, new learning may have taken place and the student needs to be enabled to link this knowledge base with practice experience. Your contract of learning will facilitate this transfer and application of knowledge. Most students will be realistic in their goals but be aware that you will meet students who want to cram too much into specific learning experiences and it is your job to guide them through his process. Ambition has to be tempered with reality! McAllister (1996) suggests that students may possess a common and irrational belief that in order to be a registered nurse a student must know about the principles of care prior to commencing practice.

Methods of assessment

As we have already seen in Chapter 4, there are a number of different methods that you can use to assess your student appropriately, both in relation to learning needs, and in respect of the learning opportunities available. On the whole, you will use direct observation to assess the practical skills of your student, and this method often demonstrates that the knowledge base on which practice is performed is present and applied. Direct observation demonstrates to you that not only can the student adequately perform some aspect of care, but that performance will demonstrate the knowledge base required for that skill. Therefore your direct observation enables you to identify and confirm that your student has applied theory to practice – you and your student have crossed the theory–practice divide!

Other methods of assessment may have been agreed between you both as appropriate to the context and reality of learning. These methods may include looking at product evidence, such as charts completed by the student, and talking to others who may have been involved in the delivery of care, such as another registered nurse, or another professional such as a physiotherapist or a social worker.

Some additional methods are:

- testimony of others

- documentation

- simulation

- case studies.

As discussed in Chapter 4, the methods of assessment and the subsequent evidence produced by the student have to be:

- valid

- reliable

- current

- authentic

- sufficient.

ACTIVITY 5.5   Identify a learning experience and list the methods of assessment you might use.

You may have identified feeding a patient, for example, and the methods of assessment might then be:

- direct observation

- questioning

- simulation.

Remember to help your student link this learning to the application of the knowledge base, for example, of the anatomy and physiology of the gastro-intestinal tract, or the concept of altered body image.

Feedback

Students need to know how they are progressing within the placement, and it is your role to give your student adequate and accurate feedback on their progress. In other words you are undertaking a formative assessment of your student. Within your learning contract you will have identified feedback and

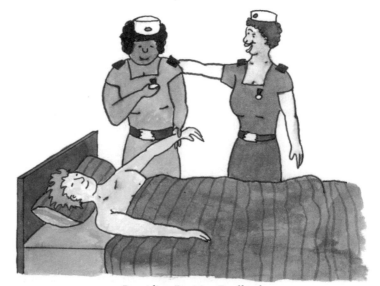

Providing Positive Feedback

review dates. These must be adhered to so that success and non-achievement can be identified, and the learning contract added to as necessary. Feedback also needs to be ongoing between the target dates. Think back to when your manager told you how good a job you were doing! It confirmed your ability, enabled you to maintain a high standard and to move your practice and learning on. Your student needs exactly the same sort of feedback, or in other terms your reflection on their learning.

Reflection

Feedback is not a one sided process and your student will be aware of the need to evaluate her own learning and achievements. Reflection is a commonly used tool and is documented in the form of reflective diaries or journals. Simplistically, reflection means 'looking back', and this is exactly what your student needs to do, matching their experiences to their objectives and learning contract. A reflective diary may contain some very personal areas, and it is up to your student to decide which parts of the diary they will share with you, and which will be kept private. This must be respected. Reflective diaries are a tool through which learning can be moved along the lifelong learning continuum.

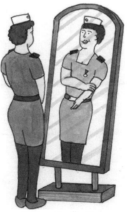

Using Reflection

CONCLUSION

The assessment of nursing students is paramount for many reasons, the main two being:

- safe and competent delivery of nursing care to all patients and clients cared for by students

- production of competent nurses who once on the NMC register act as assessors themselves, thus completing the cycle.

Although it should be implicit within all mentor/assessor practice, a word needs to be said here about the honesty and openness of mentor/assessors. Health care delivery is demanding upon time, emotions and individuals, and health care must only be delivered by competent practitioners, regardless of the status of that individual within the team. You are, through your mentor/assessor practice and decisions, responsible with others for giving 'permission' for the student to qualify and practise. This requires you to be honest, and have the courage of your convictions. If a student is not competent, you must say so. Put yourself in the patients' position: they deserve and expect competent care delivery from appropriately skilled and knowledgeable staff. The mentor/assessor role is fundamental to this!

REFERENCES

Brooker C (ed) 2001 Dictionary of nursing, 18th edn. Churchill Livingstone, Edinburgh

Dart B, Clarke J 1991 Helping students become better students: a case study in teacher education. Higher Education 22:317–35

Department of Health (DoH) 2000 A health service for all talents: developing the NHS workforce. DoH, London

Department of Health (DoH) 2001 Working together, learning together: a framework for lifelong learning for the NHS. DoH, London

English National Board and Department of Health (ENB & DoH) 2001a Placements in Focus, Guidance for education in practice for health care professions. ENB & DoH, London

English National Board and Department of Health (ENB & DoH) 2001b Preparation of mentors and teachers: a new framework of guidance. ENB & DoH 2001, London

McAllister M 1996 Learning contracts: an Australian experience. Nurse Education Today 16:199–205

Richardson S 1987 Implementing contract learning in a senior nursing practice. Journal of Advanced Nursing 12:201–6

Royal College of Nursing (RCN) 2002 Helping students get the best from their practice placements: a Royal College of Nursing toolkit. RCN, London

United Kingdom Central Council for Nursing, Midwifery and Health Visiting (UKCC) 1999 Fitness for practice: the UKCC Commission for Nursing and Midwifery Education. UKCC, London

6

Assessment: building on what you already know – AP(E)L

INTRODUCTION

As outlined earlier in this book (Ch. 3), learning is acquired in many different ways. For example, by gaining experience in particular aspects of care, from reading books, or undertaking formal modes of study, to name but a few. As nursing and midwifery education has developed there has been an increasing need to pull together some of these areas and find a way of accrediting the student with learning they have already undertaken, and in many instances that has been formally assessed previously. Many of you reading this will identify instances when you have undertaken a programme of study that contained vast amounts of material that you had learned about on an earlier course! It is clearly not in the student's best interests to cover old ground, and employers understandably do not want to support learning that has already occurred elsewhere, especially when they may have contributed towards it.

There are two main categories used within the accreditation system:

1. Accreditation of Prior Certificated Learning (APL). This involves the learning for which you have been awarded a certificate from an educational institution, e.g. college of further education, higher education or training organisation. The emphasis here is on equivalence, and it is used when there is a certificate of learning which can be verified as equal to the credit being claimed.

2. Accreditation of Prior Experiential Learning (APEL). This term is used for any uncertificated learning gained through experience. This may be in a previous job, through caring for others in an informal way or voluntary work. APEL is used where the learning has not involved formal courses but can be verified. 'APEL is very important as it is what a person can do and knows rather than the courses he/she has attended which is important (Woolhouse et al 2001, p. 112).

Taken together, as a system within which students are awarded credit, they are identified as Accreditation of Prior and Experiential Learning, or AP(E)L.

Anyone can use AP(E)L within their learning. This could mean you as a trainee mentor looking for credit for previous experience – e.g. City & Guilds 730 programme: Preparation of Teacher Certificate level. Or it could include a student nurse or HCA on placement with you who is seeking credit for experience gained elsewhere – e.g. an S/NVQ level 3 candidate who already has S/NVQ level 2 credits, or a nursing student at the end of the branch programme with identified and assessed learning. This chapter is for mentors/assessors applying for credit from assessment of skills or any other programme of learning. However the principles applied in this chapter are relevant to all learners and you are encouraged to apply the principles to your individual situation.

The purpose of this chapter therefore, is to provide you with an understanding of the AP(E)L system, and how you can benefit from the process whilst at the same time recognising the pitfalls.

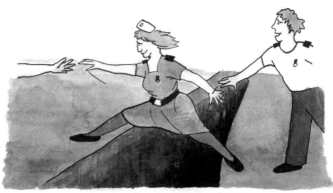

Overcoming the Pitfalls of APEL

LEARNING OBJECTIVES

After reading this chapter you should be able to:

◆ explain the accreditation system relating to nursing and midwifery education

◆ understand the processes involved in accreditation

◆ identify the factors to be considered when applying for accreditation

◆ understand how to put together your profile for accreditation

◆ recognise the different university systems of accreditation.

ATTEMPTING DEFINITIONS

Rickards (1992, p. 28) provides a very straightforward definition of both prior learning and accreditation: 'prior learning is what you already know how to do, and accreditation is finding an appropriate way to give you credit for it'. In essence, prior learning is recognised by the accumulation of credit and transferred to another area or programme of study. You are then accredited with that learning. Initially there appear to be more questions than answers:

● how do you know what you know?

● what is an appropriate way of being given credit?

● what is a level of study?

● how do we know you have reached it and who says so?

Toyne (1979) describes the system of credit accumulation and transfer as a scheme whereby qualifications, part qualifications and learning experiences are given appropriate recognition or credit to enable students to progress their studies without necessarily having to repeat materials or levels of study. You may be forgiven at this stage for wondering why anyone would want to enter the potentially largely confusing credit accumulation and transfer system, and certainly some difficulties have been identified. There is much anecdotal evidence about students who have found it impossible to transfer credit between one university and another, but if certain procedures and processes are followed the process can run quite smoothly.

THE HISTORY OF AP(E)L

The move of nursing and midwifery education into the higher education sector has enabled the profession to become much more integrated into the field of education generally. As a result it has been able to benefit from some of the flexible processes available relating to learning, for example modular approaches to education and the ability to use prior learning as a building block for further areas of study. The move has also meant that the systems that now drive nursing and midwifery education fall into university structures, e.g. quality measurement tools discussed in Chapter 1. Additionally, as a practice based profession we learn a vast amount of skills and knowledge over time. As nursing and nursing care have changed and developed, so too have your skills.

It is interesting to note, however, that informal accreditation of prior learning is not new to nursing and midwifery. Some kind of accreditation of prior learning has always been carried out at important points of transition. 'All tests and examinations that determine whether an individual can be awarded a particular qualification or whether they can proceed to the next stage of the system are ways of accrediting prior learning' (Rickards 1992, p. 28). An extremely good example of this is the need for nursing students to complete a common foundation programme successfully before being able to progress to the branch. In theory at least, students are able to be accredited with the common foundation programme and on successful completion should be able to undertake the branch at any university offering the same preregistration qualification.

The Welsh National Board clearly placed AP(E)L in the context of nursing and nurses' professional development with the following definition: 'AP(E)L refers to the formal acknowledgement of an individual's previous learning and experiences so that academic credit may be awarded, thus avoiding repetition and maximising flexible approaches to continuing professional development'.

APPLYING FOR ACCREDITATION

The first question to ask yourself is why you want to apply for accreditation. This question may seem rather obvious but it is essential that accreditation is looked at not only as a paper collection exercise, and completing an award earlier than the allotted time, but also in terms of what it will actually mean to you as an individual. It is clear that nurses and midwives, with their development of knowledge and skills gained in practice, are excellent candidates for accreditation but this must be harnessed in some way. This leads us to the issue of why we cannot simply be accredited with what we know by virtue of the length of our experience, and why it is necessary for universities and the NMC to make sure that what we have learned is properly assessed. The emphasis on professional development for nurses and midwives (NMC 2002a) places upon us the requirement to continually develop our skills and knowledge as opposed to collecting individual certificates. It is obviously helpful if both of these aspects fit together since this may prove to be important for career development. Essentially it is how what we have learned will influence patient care rather than the paper award at the end of it. These principles identified above are clearly reflected in the document *Preparation of mentors and teachers* (ENB & DoH 2001) which provides contemporary guidance for the development of mentor and teacher preparation programmes (discussed in Chs 4 and 5).

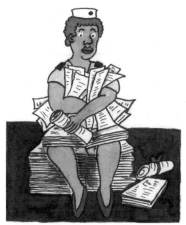

More than a Paper Exercise!

Building on past experience

A major building block for any accreditation is being comfortable with what you already know. Only then can you begin to fill the gaps.

ACTIVITY 6.1   Take a few minutes to jot down some of the skills you have learned purely by being at work either in the ward, a patient's home, health centre or clinic.

Time permitting and depending on how long you have been doing your current work you could probably fill a large notebook! Why then should this learning not be recognised and parts of it used as a basis for further learning?

There are however some potential disadvantages to this. Universities are autonomous. For example, think about the different criteria that universities require for entry into preregistration nursing and midwifery programmes. Some will accept minimum requirements whilst others raise the stakes. This means that their awards of credit are also likely to be different. So just because you have undertaken a module in a specific subject does not necessarily mean you would be accredited with that module if you decided to change university in mid programme. In addition, universities may well have different 'ceilings' of how much prior learning they are willing to permit credit for. This can range from anything between 20% and 60% of a course. Again, some universities award a maximum amount of credit for the type of programme awarded. For example 30 credits for a postgraduate certificate, 60 credits for a postgraduate diploma and 80 credits for a masters programme.

With this in mind it is obvious that applying for credit is not necessarily an easy option. It does however, send out a very clear message if you are embarking on the accreditation pathway: make sure that you have a full understanding of your particular university's rules about the maximum credit to which you would be entitled.

PRINCIPLES UNDERPINNING THE ACCREDITATION PROCESS

There may be some slight differences in the accreditation process depending on the individual university involved. The University of Manchester (1999) identifies seven key principles:

1. Where credits are given, they should be given for learning, not for experience alone. (The message here is that you must be able to demonstrate what you have learned rather than just what you know.)

2. Credits may be given for prior learning, where the level, standard, content, relevance and currency of that learning are appropriate to a particular programme of study. (It is very unlikely that any university

will give you credit on the basis of a certificate you undertook some 20 years ago. It is better to say what you learned as a result of it.)

3. The maximum number of credits which may be awarded is 80 for a masters programme, 60 for a postgraduate diploma and 30 for a postgraduate certificate.

4. AP(E)L has to be based on consistent principles of academic judgement.

5. No AP(E)L award may be given which implies partial completion of a course unit. Credit can only be given for whole course units.

6. It is the student's responsibility to prepare an application and submit adequate documentation. Guidance and counselling may be sought from the university where appropriate.

7. A student must apply for credit exemption before registering on a programme.

In short, the responsibility for applying for credit always rests with you and not with the university to which you are applying.

> The responsibility for attempting to gain accreditation rests firmly on you, the individual candidate. Ultimately you must make a claim for accreditation supported with acceptable evidence (in the form of a portfolio). Making a claim involves seeking help from an appropriate lecturer or teacher in a college or educational establishment approved to conduct the AP(E)L process. The teacher will then provide detailed explanation of the process and the tasks and standards to be undertaken and met. This constitutes the learning contract.

The need for rigour in the accreditation process

ACTIVITY 6.2

In relation to the profession of nursing and midwifery there are many reasons why the process needs to be rigorous. Make a list of the reasons why you think it necessary that any prior learning you have undertaken is formally assessed in this way.

Hopefully at the very top of your list, will be patient/client safety. It is obvious that if courses are to be passed successfully then the institution responsible for giving the award meets the criteria for public safety. In nursing and midwifery these are set down by the NMC and form part of the Quality Frameworks for courses of study as outlined in Chapter 2. You may also have some of the following reasons on your list as identified by Atkins (1993):

- to establish the level of achievement reached at the end of a course, or the *progress made during a course*
- to give a recognition by making awards or assigning credit
- to diagnose students strengths weaknesses and gaps in their learning in order *that remedial action can be taken*
- to motivate students and stimulate further reading
- to predict a student's likely performance in the future for purposes of selection or *progression*
- to select for employment
- to ensure requirements of external regulatory bodies (e.g. the NMC) are met
- to help teaches and mentors improve their performance and to improve the *conditions for learning by providing feedback*
- to determine the extent to which course aims or intended learning outcomes have *been achieved*.

THE ADVANTAGES AND DISADVANTAGES OF MAKING AN APPLICATION

There are clearly many advantages in applying, but as previously mentioned the value of the application rests with you as an individual weighing up some of the advantages and disadvantages.

ACTIVITY 6.3   Make a list of advantages and disadvantages to help you decide whether it is the best course of action for you.

You may have identified some of the following advantages:

- early completion of the course you are undertaking
- avoidance of going over old ground
- may work out cheaper (may not depending on the university system used)
- may enable you to focus purely on what you want to learn as opposed to the full curriculum.

And some disadvantages:

- may feel detached from your peer group

- may not feel confident that you know enough to be accredited

- may feel isolated if other students are all going through the same modules.

It is important to remember that no student has to undertake the AP(E)L process – even if you have relevant experience, it is largely up to you to decide whether or not to apply. If you decide to enter the accreditation system, the following is designed to give you an overview of the systems and processes involved.

ACCREDITATION SYSTEMS USED IN HIGHER EDUCATION

Higher education institutions operate what is known as a credit accumulation and transfer scheme or CATS scheme for short. This is the system used for placing and awarding credit upon study you have previously undertaken. Its strength is that it enables you to obtain some exemption towards qualification or award by gaining credit for the different courses of study and areas of learning that you have already successfully completed or undertaken. This may include the award of credits for a course of study or professional experience as a nurse, midwife or health visitor. Generally, higher education courses begin with credit points offered at three academic levels:

- level 1, equivalent to certificate level (e.g. nurses undertaking training prior to preregistration nursing courses)

- level 2, equivalent to a diploma (Diploma in nursing or health studies)

- level 3, equivalent to a bachelor degree (BSc in Nursing).

There are differences across the 4 countries of the UK. For example, Scotland awards SCOTCATS. Universities tend to adopt two distinct areas for accreditation:

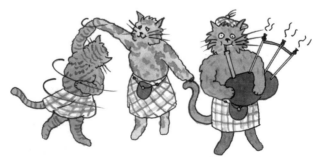

Credit Accumulation and Transfer in Scotland

1. General accreditation. This relates to study that has been undertaken at a particular academic level. A good example is someone who wants to undertake a degree in nursing who has already gained a degree in sociology. The student will already have learned the analytical skills required at degree level and as a result these are transferable to another programme of study.

2. Specific accreditation. This is awarded where previous learning relates directly to the study you wish to undertake. For example, in relation to nursing this could be in pharmaceuticals or counselling, ethics or communication skills.

To clarify, specific credit points are awarded for exemption from particular courses. General credit points are awarded for achievements which may not be directly related to the course of study for which you are seeking credit, but may be seen as demonstrating ability and as such are transferable.

THINKING ABOUT YOUR CLAIM

Students applying for AP(E)L will be assessed at different levels and you must prepare your evidence to take account of this and be aware of what institutions are looking for in order to be accredited with an area of learning. As mentioned, universities begin their accreditation process at level 1, equivalent to certificate level. All of us who became registered nurses prior to the implementation of Project 2000 were accredited at this level. Level 2 equates with diploma, as with the majority of preregistration education programmes. Level 3 equates to bachelor degree. It is important to note however that increasingly some preregistration education programmes are being pitched at advanced diploma level and as a result carry some level 3 points.

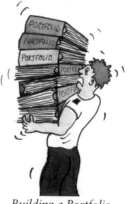

Building a Portfolio

In general terms to be awarded credit at level 1 you will need to provide evidence that you have both knowledge and understanding of the subject for which you require credit, and equally importantly that you can apply that knowledge and understanding to the care you provide as a nurse. The following gives a very rough guide as to the criteria that may be used when looking for evidence at the three academic levels. It would however be prudent to ask your individual university for its particular criteria and guidance.

In general, level 1 criteria demand that:

- the evidence provides a clear understanding of the issues and concepts and their relationships

- the material presented is accurate and relevant to the area of study

- the material is logically presented and demonstrates evidence of reading of the subject

- the evidence demonstrates application of the material to practice.

At Level 2 the candidate must:

- be able to demonstrate the ability to analyse and reflect on key issues

- demonstrate reflective application of theory and practice

- ensure arguments are well organised

- give evidence of concluding arguments

- show clear evidence of wider reading

- demonstrate critical understanding of the literature.

To be accredited at level 2 you will need to be able to demonstrate what is happening as a result of the knowledge and understanding you have gained. Can you demonstrate how the knowledge you have gained has enabled you to solve specific problems?

Level 3 requires:

- demonstration of analysis, synthesis and reflection

- theory and practice to be clearly integrated

- the utilisation of relevant research

- that relevant and appropriate research/theories are consistently applied to the material presented

- that it is appropriately referenced

- that presentation of work is legible and grammatically correct, including good use of language

- that arguments are well organised with evidence of wide reading demonstrated by depth and breadth of knowledge

- the ability to analyse and incorporate theories concepts and principles to the practice of nursing

- ability to demonstrate how the material presented contributes to the practice of nursing

- the ability to analyse own assumptions, values and ideas in constructive argument

- the ability to assess the strengths and weaknesses of the points of the argument presented.

The emphasis here is on analysis, change and evaluation. It is not just knowing about a certain subject, but being able to dissect it. You need to ask yourself how you have changed your practice as a result of what you have learned and what difference it has made to the patients/clients in your care or the colleagues with whom you work.

ACTIVITY 6.4   Try to think of an example of past learning that would fit these criteria.

Finding out what you need to know

Accreditation is without doubt an individual process and it is important to recognise that the evidence you provide is yours alone. Whilst others may be able to provide support, your evidence must reflect your individual learning. As a result the questions you would wish to ask will also be different.

ACTIVITY 6.5   Make a list of what you would want to know from an institution if you wish to gain credit from previous study.

You will probably list some questions similar to the following:

- Why do I want to apply for credit?

- What evidence do I have to present in support of my claim?

- What are the learning outcomes of the course for which I wish to apply for credit, and what aspects of my past learning and experience match them?
- What process will be used to decide whether my previous learning is acceptable?
- How much will it cost?
- How long will it take?
- Is it acceptable to the NMC as part of my professional development?
- What evidence of my previous learning is required?
- At what stage in my study will I be accredited with my previous learning?

Knowing what you already know and putting your claim together

Putting together a claim for AP(E)L should, in theory at least, be easier than in previous years largely because we should all by now have a profile of learning as part of NMC requirements in relation to PREP. Whilst the purpose of portfolios for accreditation and to meet the requirements of the NMC are fundamentally different, using the NMC (2002b) guidelines is as useful a place as any to begin developing your portfolio. Definitions of portfolios are given in Chapter 5.

ACTIVITY 6.6   Try to think of the reasons why the requirements of a university looking to accredit you with prior learning may be different from what the NMC is looking for in order to maintain your registration.

Universities tend to look for evidence of depth of knowledge in your learning that matches a course or programme of study they are currently offering. They therefore need to know specifically that you have met the outcomes for that course. On the other hand, the NMC's main focus is on ensuring that as a registered nurse, midwife or health visitor you meet the two PREP standards set by them:

1. PREP practice standard – you must have worked in some capacity by virtue of your nursing or midwifery qualification during the previous 5 years for a minimum of 100 days (750 hours) or have successfully undertaken an approved return to practice course.

2. PREP (continuing professional development) standard – you must have undertaken and recorded your continuing professional development

(CPD) over the 3 years prior to the renewal of your registration demonstrating a minimum of 35 hours over the intervening 3-year reregistration period. All registered nurses and midwives have been required to comply with this standard since April 1995. Since April 2000, registrants need to have declared on their notification of practice form that they have met this requirement when they renew their registration (NMC 2002b).

There are many books and articles available that will take you through the steps of building your portfolio, e.g. McGrother (1995) and Nganasurian (1999), so it is intended just to give you the key pointers here. A good base-line to work from is to write your portfolio assuming that whoever reads and assesses it does not know you and has never met you in their life. It is sad but true that in many assessments the student assumes that the teacher already knows what the student knows, and as a result fails to provide the appropriate information. McGrother (1995) provides a very useful framework:

- Start the first page with who you are and where you work including name, PIN number, work address, home address and telephone number.

- Page 2 should include a list of all your professional and academic qualifications in chronological order.

However, to meet NMC standards and to start to develop your portfolio, you cannot stop there. What is crucial in this exercise is to identify what you have learned from undertaking the qualification you have been awarded. So for example you may at some time in your life have undertaken a computer literacy course, but what exactly did you learn and how have you been able to use this in the work you are now undertaking? To continue with this example, it may be that you learned how to undertake a literature search and you are now able to use this when looking for evidence to enhance your nursing practice. This you need to write down as evidence.

McGrother (1995) suggests using the following 'headers' for each piece of study whether it be a conference you have attended, a study day, meeting or course:

- subject of course, meeting, etc., e.g. moving and handling

- validating body, e.g. university course, study day by employer

- what it was that you learned

- how you have used the learning in your work

- how you will develop your portfolio further.

It is important to note here that what you learn in areas other than formal study is equally as valid, particularly in meeting NMC standards of practice. So for example, you can learn from reading articles on your particular area of practice, discussing with colleagues or undertaking visits to other areas. How your learning has influenced your practice is key. As identified in Chapter 5, reflection is the main method for achieving this.

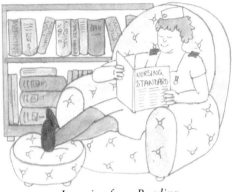

Learning from Reading

Some specific questions you might like to consider when you are reflecting on your learning from experience might be:

- What was your school experience like?

- What paid employment experiences have you had?

- What unpaid employment experiences have you had?

- Have you undertaken any voluntary work?

- What are your interest/leisure activities?

- What activities have you taken responsibility for and organised?

- Why did you decide to apply for this course?

On completion, the key questions are:

- After checking your plan, reflective commentary and evidence, consider whether your claim is valid. Have you met all of the learning outcomes for entry or credit?

- Is the evidence sufficient proof for entry to the modules you are claiming?

- Is the evidence current?

- Is the direct evidence your own work?

You should include all relevant activities you have attended, organised or assisted with, for example:

- courses and modules
- conferences
- study days
- journals/articles
- project work
- debates/seminars
- participation in journal clubs
- participation in quality circles
- participation in induction programmes
- supervision and assessment activities
- critical incidents
- research activities
- practical experience
- open learning materials.

Other activities, which you may wish to utilise as a means of gaining credit for learning, might include elements of your non-professional experience. For example, if you belong to or chair the local parent and teacher association, then you may be able to describe this type of activity in a manner which could count as evidence of organisational skills learning. An individual who has worked with Samaritans or in other voluntary capacities may be able to make a credible claim for communication or counselling skills. Even some recreational activities may be eligible for inclusion, such as captaining a sports team or writing short commentaries on local issues for local newspapers.

A FRAMEWORK FOR YOUR APPLICATION

Rickards (1992) identifies six phases in the AP(E)L process which provide a useful framework if you are planning on making an application:

1. Pre-entry. The pre-entry phase relates to you as the candidate deciding what particular areas of study you wish to undertake and what areas of

knowledge and skills you have that could be accredited. It also involves getting the right sort of advice in order to put your claim together.

2. Candidate profiling. This requires you to think about those areas of your previous study that you may wish to submit for accreditation. The easiest way of doing this is to look at the outcomes for the course or module you wish to be accredited against and ask yourself whether you have met those outcomes through previous study or experience.

3. Gathering evidence. This involves pulling together all the information you have about your learning specific to the claim. In addition to recognised certificates, this could involve for example your reflections on critical incidents and evidence of how your practice had changed.

4. Assessment. This relates to the submission of your evidence and your receipt of a clear understanding of the path your application will take and the expected time required to undertake the assessment.

5. Accreditation. This involves the formal acknowledgement of your accreditation.

6. Post assessment guidance. This reminds you to seek guidance not only if your application requires further work but also to clarify what the accreditation implies, should your application be successful, in relation to any further study.

SOME DO'S AND DON'TS WHEN MAKING AN AP(E)L CLAIM

The following advice is adapted from McGrother (1995).

Always ask at the college where you wish to make a claim before getting down to any intensive work. Friends mean to be helpful, but just because they have successfully been accredited with prior learning, it does not follow that you will automatically be successful, even if you have undertaken the same course. This is because it is what you have learned that is crucial to the process rather than the piece of paper you have been awarded as a result of it. A great deal of extra work and heartache can be avoided at this point. Always ask for help from the university. It is perfectly right and proper for you to request guidance at each stage of your evidence collection, otherwise how will you know if you are on the right track. If help is not forthcoming do you need to consider whether it is the right university at which to be undertaking your studies?

Don't fall into the trap of telling the assessor everything you know about the subject for which you wish to be accredited. Page after page of explanation will not demonstrate how you have used your knowledge in practice. Make sure at your tutorials that your evidence is at the appropriate level for which you are making a claim. Make sure your experience is relevant.

It is a common but inaccurate assumption that the assessment of portfolios is largely a subjective exercise undertaken by one particular teacher. It is, however, important to be aware that your portfolio is assessed against a preordained set of criteria, not at the whim of an assessor, so it is crucial that you meet these. In addition, portfolios are often assessed by teams of assessors with access to an external examiner whose role is to ensure the criteria are applied consistently and fairly.

WHAT HAPPENS TO YOUR CLAIM?

Following submission of your claim it will be assessed against the university's criteria, which is why it is essential to get the appropriate help and advice from someone within the university at the start to ensure you meet their particular guidelines. A word of caution here. Never submit any portfolio – the same goes for essays and projects – without first getting a receipt. This is not because the university is in any way unscrupulous, but purely because in all areas of life things get lost. It is impossible to accredit anyone with something that has not been seen. By the same token and for the same reasons always photocopy anything that lends itself to photocopying.

Expect a cost for accessing the AP(E)L system. This varies between institutions and it is possible for different charges to be made depending on whether your application for credit is for experiential or prior learning. Some universities may also charge you on a sliding scale, i.e. the more credits you apply for, the greater the cost. It is obviously very important that you ask this question at the very first stage. Clearly you would not embark on buying a car without ascertaining the cost. Buying accreditation is no different in principle.

CONCLUSION

The road to receiving credit for prior learning in nursing is neither straight nor narrow. It requires a great deal of time effort and understanding of the processes involved before even embarking on it, although undoubtedly the more you become involved the more expert you will become.

In real life you do not set out on a journey without knowing where you are heading, and in this respect accreditation is no different. It is crucial to plan the route and have a list of appropriate questions at the ready in case you get lost.

REFERENCES

Atkins M 1993: cited in Assessing and accrediting work based learning. www.dfes.gov.uk/heqe/wblchp7.htm

English National Board and Department of Health (ENB & DoH) 2001 Preparation of mentors and teachers: a new framework for guidance. ENB & DoH, London

McGrother J 1995 Profiles, portfolios and how to build them. Scutari Press, London

Nganasurian W 1999 Accreditation of prior learning for nurses and midwives. Quay Books, Dinton

Nursing and Midwifery Council (NMC) 2002a Code of professional conduct. NMC, London

Nursing and Midwifery Council (NMC) 2002b The PREP handbook. NMC, London

Rickards T 1992 How to win as a mature student. Kogan Page, London

Toyne P 1979 Educational credit transfer: feasibility study. DES, London

University of Manchester 1999 Academic Standards Code of Practice. Available online at www.search.mcc.ac.uk/cgi-bin/htsearch

Woolhouse M, Jones T, Rees M 2001 Teaching the post-16 learner. Northcote House, Tavistock

FURTHER READING

Nganasurian W 1999 Accreditation of prior learning for nurses and midwives. Quay Books, Dinton. A very comprehensive and easy-to-read book on APL. It gives clear practical advice on preparing and submitting your claim whilst at the same time guiding you through the processes used in its implementation.

Glossary

Accreditation   The process used in educational settings to recognise and make an award for previous learning.

AMA (Advanced Modern Apprenticeships)   Schemes and awards which incorporate NVQs, key skills and technical certificates at NVQ level 3 (see FMA).

CATS (Credit Accumulation and Transfer Scheme)   The system used in higher education to credit students for learning they have previously undertaken.

Certificated learning   Learning which has resulted in a certificate of achievement.

Chronological   According to sequence of time.

Commentary   A piece of writing in which the writer gives an opinion, e.g. on another person's work or an event or occurrence.

CPD (Continuing Professional Development)   Learning undertaken following preregistration education that increases the nurse's knowledge and skills thus improving patient/client care.

Credit accumulation   The building up of credit from previous certificated or experiential learning.

Devolution   The transfer of business from a central body, e.g. central government to local government, RCN governance to RCN Boards and regions.

Experiential learning   Learning that has been acquired from work.

FMA (Foundation Modern Apprenticeship)   Schemes and awards covering NVQs, key skills and technical certificates at NVQ level 2 (see AMAs).

HCA (Health Care Assistant)   A term usually denoting an individual working to support professionals, e.g. nurses, and usually undertaking S/NVQ awards. Often used synonymously with other titles such as Health Care Support Worker (HCSW), nursing auxiliary, nursing assistant, care assistant.

Perception   The way in which we come to understand what is happening around us by interpreting what is happening in ourselves and our surroundings, using expectations, experience and senses.

PDP (Personal Development Plan)   A plan of development formulated by an individual, usually with the support and input of the manager to identify learning needs over short and long term settings. May be used in an appraisal system, and registered nurses may use these alongside their portfolios of evidence used for PREP needs.

PIN (Personal Identification Number)   The unique number given to an individual on registration with the NMC, which remains unchanged throughout their continuous registration. This number is noted on the 'credit card' received every 3 years upon re-registration with the NMC.

PREP (Post Registration Education and Practice)   The system in place to ensure nurses, midwives and health visitors meet the appropriate standards to practise.

NCVQ (National Council for Vocational Qualifications)   Was the regulatory body for NVQs, now subsumed into the QCA.

NOS (National Occupational Standards)   The units of competence which, grouped together, form S/NVQ awards.

OS (Occupational Standards)   Standards used to describe the intended outcomes of specific roles/professions.

QCA (Qualifications and Curriculum Authority)   Successor to the NCVQ, a much larger organisation regulating a variety of educational issues, e.g. GCSE and A-level, as well as NVQs.

SCOTCATS   The system used in higher education in Scotland to credit students with learning they have previously undertaken.

S/NVQ (Scottish and National Vocational Qualifications)   Qualifications developed by a sector for a sector, e.g. the vast healthcare system includes and involves public, private and independent stakeholders.

SSB (Standard Setting Body)   An organisation that sets standards, usually NOSs (see above) for a particular sector or industry. For example, Skills for Health is the SSB for the health sector.

Index